Human Nutrition

R. F. Mottram MB BS BSc PhD

Senior Lecturer in Physiology, University College, Cardiff

Edward Arnold

© R. F. Mottram 1979

First published 1948
Edward Arnold (Publishers) Ltd.,
41 Bedford Square, London WC1B 3DQ
Reprinted 1951, 1954 (with amendments), 1957, 1960
Second edition 1963
Reprinted in paperback with amendments 1972
Reprinted 1974, 1976
Third edition 1979
Reprinted 1981

British Library Cataloguing Publication Data
Mottram, R F
   Human nutrition.—3rd ed.
   1. Nutrition
   I. Title   II. Mottram, Roy Frederick
   641.1   TX353

   ISBN 0-7131-4331-2

Phototypeset in V.I.P. Plantin by
Western Printing Services Ltd, Bristol
Printed in Great Britain by
Pitman Press Ltd, Bath

Preface

People need food, and cannot live for long without eating enough of it. By enough, I mean some hundreds of grams of solid material containing the right amounts of many different chemical substances. In most human societies food comes from agricultural processes, and one can safely say that civilisation is based on agriculture, its whole complex structure supported on this one foundation. If its agriculture is unsound in practice or product, sooner or later that civilisation will fall.

The knowledge of the right sort of food for man and how it may best be brought to his table—the science of nutrition—is a product mainly of the twentieth century. The previous fifty years had seen some increase in knowledge of our needs for energy and for protein and we had begun deliberately to interfere with raw foodstuffs in our infant chemical industry in order to overcome shortages, preserve foods better, and to present them for consumption in a more palatable form. In the first forty years of this century there came a sudden vast extension of knowledge of our nutritional needs with the discovery of vitamins and their role in our internal chemistry, the study of functions of the individual amino acids of proteins, and of our needs for various organic and inorganic substances, many only in pin-head quantities. Then in recent decades, we have had cause to suspect that some diseases (in addition to the various deficiency diseases) may be aggravated or caused partially by eating too much of the wrong food.

Knowledge of the human aspect of nutrition, how much of each material each one of us needs each day, has developed in parallel with knowledge of how to produce, preserve and prepare foodstuffs for human consumption, and knowledge on both fronts is still developing. Nutrition is a young science. New facts are continually being discovered and the explanation and interpretation of these, and their integration into the body of knowledge that is nutrition continually proceeds. Already by the 1940s, the science was sufficiently advanced for British Government Food Policy in the second world war to improve the average person's nutritional status and his health.

The real advances of the subject have been made by biochemists, physiologists, chemists, agricultural scientists and by medical practitioners and professional dietitians. Often the research findings are hidden in the pages of scientific journals, not readily accessible to the general public and written in an exotic jargon understood only by the expert! The need exists to collect and interpret these correctly for the ordinary person, in language that he can easily understand, and without evoking his fear of the unknown. We need also to avoid the flashing eye and the strident voice of the man with the message, crying 'woe unto ye (unless you follow my own particular set pathway to safety)!' We need to translate correctly the language of science into terms of milk, cheese, meat, eggs, bread, vegetables and fruit, and to know how cooking and food preserving may conserve or destroy the value of the foods we eat. In this translation the quality of 'scientific objectivity' must be preserved. The place of a book such as this is to explain and to teach, and not to arouse emotions or to preach.

This book is being offered as a primer in the spread of knowledge of nutrition, and should serve as an introduction only to the complex subjects set out in more ambitious volumes on nutrition. I view the subject primarily as a physiologist, concerned with all aspects of how the living human body works. I will consider nutrition objectively, that is, without prejudice or emotion, though I will admit to two prejudices. One is that I am against prejudice itself in others, and the other is that food should be produced and distributed to all people *as a right* of those people, and not at the whim or to the financial gain of private individuals. Equally the rights of the producers themselves must be protected and finally we must guarantee that food production methods employed today do not harm the potential of the earth to produce the food that our children's children will need. Although the subject of this last prejudice of mine is largely beyond the scope of this book, I hope that you, the reader, will continually bear it in mind as you think about how best to translate 'nutritional requirements' into the food you buy and eat. You should remember, too, the sorts of repercussions one agricultural development may have on many other practices. Thus, after the second world war, the need to produce more milk safely in Great Britain led to electricity being taken to many remote moorland valleys, an increase in their cattle stocks, improvement in fertility and hay crops of the valley fields, increase in the number of sheep that could be over-wintered, and a great change in the social life of the people of the valleys. Abundant milk, lamb and wool were obtained, but imported cattle-feed concentrates had to be found from abroad with many economic and social consequences for many people in different parts of the earth.

In producing this, the third edition of this book, I am following in the footsteps of my father, the late Professor V. H. Mottram. It could be truthfully said that he pioneered the teaching of nutrition, both to his students at King's College of Household and Social Science (now Queen Elizabeth College) in London, and to the general public in many newspaper articles and wireless talks in the 1920s and 1930s. I hope that in this edition I can reach the same high standard that he achieved in presenting the facts and theories of nutrition to you, the reader. Like him I must acknowledge the permission of the Controller of HM Stationery Office, and of the authors, for the use of the tables in *The Composition of Foods* by McCance and Widdowson. I would also like to record the help and advice I have received from many in producing this volume. I must thank Mrs Tina Harris for her work in deciphering my handwriting and preparing the typescript for the publishers and Mr Hywel Bines for preparing the spirometer figure.

Many thanks are also due to the authors of *Human Nutrition and Dietetics* for permission to include tables of vitamin contents of foods, to Churchill-Livingstone, publishers of the book, and to Blackwell Scientific Publications for permission to reproduce the figure of the new Palmer Spirometer (Fig. 5.3).

R. F. Mottram
Thetford and Cardiff, 1977

Contents

1
The science of nutrition

The science of nutrition is the body of knowledge of the foods a living organism requires, how they may be produced, how the organism uses the foods and how it deals with the waste products.

All living beings grow and reproduce themselves, and sustain themselves in an internal state of 'dynamic equilibrium' which is frequently far removed from the true static equilibrium state of a non-living physicochemical entity. To perform these activities they take in food materials from the outside world, treat them chemically, extract energy from them and convert some of the foodstuffs into their own substance. Some of the food eaten will not be absorbable and has to be excreted from the body at the anus. The remainder, after absorption, undergoes various changes, collectively referred to as *metabolism*. Some of these result in growth and repair of tissues and are termed *anabolic* processes. In others, the foodstuffs (or body tissues and storage materials) are broken down, usually to obtain energy. This is called *catabolism*. *Exogenous* catabolism is the breaking down of foodstuffs as soon as they have been absorbed into the body, and *endogenous* catabolism is the breaking down of materials that had previously, in *anabolism*, been incorporated into the body's tissues. In practice, it is often not possible to distinguish between exogenous and endogenous catabolism, though the balance between the two processes becomes of great importance in studying both metabolism and nutrition of proteins, and in the dietary control of weight—a subject of concern to many.

Green plants obtain their food from the inorganic soluble substances found in the soil, from water and from carbon dioxide in the air. They obtain energy directly from sunlight. The trapping of this energy enables plants to build up, from sunlight and inorganic compounds, the vast array of the chemical substances that plants contain, many of them carrying in their molecules some of the energy of the sunlight that was so essential in their formation. Whether it be duckweed floating on a pond surface, or a giant redwood tree, all plants depend upon the same simple chemicals and upon sunlight for their food, and nutrition of plants is concerned with seeing that these substances are present in the soil or air in the amounts they require.

Animals either use green plants for their food, being what we call *herbivorous*, e.g. cattle, sheep, deer, or they eat other animals, and are described as *carnivorous*, e.g. lion, dog, seal or eagle.

Some animals are more adaptable than the strict herbivore or carnivore. Domestic dogs or even cats will eat considerable quantities of vegetable foods. Rats and pigs will eat anything, but man is one of the most adaptable of animals! The primitive hominids from before the Ice Age were carnivorous, though the use of tools meant that the powerful jaws and large canine teeth of other carnivorous animals did not evolve in our hominid ancestry. Our guts, though, are typically carnivorous in structure and function and it can be argued that some of the ills of modern man are caused by our eating excessive amounts of food of vegetable origin, such as sugar. Some human races are healthy upon a purely carnivorous diet and others on an almost completely herbivorous diet, but I take strong exception to those vegetarians who assert that it is 'unnatural' for man to eat meat!

In this book we will be dealing with the average *omnivorous* man (that is, one who will eat anything), with the sources of the various materials he needs and with the nutrient content of the various foods he eats. We will trace the foods into his body and see how they are handled there, with their anabolism and catabolism and the removal of their waste products. We will look briefly at some of the social and economic aspects that govern what we eat and at some of the more personal psychological factors concerned. We will also consider the subject of dietetics.

Dietetics has been defined as 'the interpretation and application of the hitherto discovered scientific principles of nutrition to the human subject in health and disease'. The emphasis on the words 'hitherto discovered' should serve to remind the student that nutrition, as a fundamental science, is always growing and changing and that dietetics must grow and change also. What may be taught as truth today will become error in a year or a decade. Thus it used to be taught that a fixed daily intake of vitamins of the B-group were needed for the proper utilisation of the carbohydrate content (starch and sugar) of the food. Today it is realised that the bacteria of the intestine make some of these, in varying amounts and they can be absorbed when the bacteria release them into the intestinal contents. The amount of these vitamins needed in the food is thus unknown, but will vary from person to person and in the same person at different times. Alterations in dietary habits are known to alter intestinal bacteria, as do many of the antibiotic medicines. The application of this knowledge to dietetics is that the nutritional requirements so emphatically stated on breakfast cereal packets are probably not absolutely true. Another example stems from studies of anaemia which in the earlier years of this century was frequently due to a diet deficient in iron. Wheat bran and spinach have a high iron content so it was at one time stated that to include these foods in the diet would reduce anaemia. It was found in 1937 for spinach and in 1942 for wheat bran that this iron is not available to the human body, for these foods also contain materials, oxalic acid and *phytic acid*, respectively which combine firmly with the iron and prevents its absorption from the intestine. In applying the scientific principles of nutrition to the human subject and his actual food intake, it is not sufficient to apply the principles known when the dietitian was trained. The body of knowledge in nutrition will have changed in, say, three years and the practice of dietetics must be changed in step with it. This is, of course, true in every science, but especially true in a rapidly developing science such as nutrition. A further warning, though, must be given. The latest discovery is always emphasised (especially by its discoverer!) out of relation to its true significance in the whole body of knowledge. Because 'fibre' is low in diets where diabetes is common, it does not *necessarily* follow that diabetes is a disease due to fibre deficiency or that one can cure the disease by adding fibre to the patient's diet.

Research in nutrition proceeds in biochemical, physiological, medical and agricultural (both plant and animal rearing) laboratories throughout the world. Observations made in abnormal conditions, such as where droughts produce starvation, or where a population moves into a different social environment with different foods available, add extensively to our knowledge of nutrition, as do those in special closed communities, or in groups or individual people who have acquired unusual eating habits. In some way the practising dietitian has got to continue to be aware of the advances in nutritional knowledge throughout his or her professional life. 'Dietitians' fall roughly into three categories.

The hospital dietitian

This person's function is to translate the doctor's dietary prescriptions into attractive dishes for his patient. Such a person must not only have a knowledge and understanding of dietetics and/or nutrition (and its foundations in chemistry and physiology), but must also understand the alterations in bodily function that occur in human disease and either be a good cook or have a thorough understanding of cooking methods. Since the patient must be willing to eat the food, the dietitian must consult the patient's likes and dislikes and encourage him to accept the diet prescribed. Thus, at all times, the therapeutic dietitian is working with sick people, and is in constant contact with them, just as are the other members of the therapeutic professional team. She is thus *in no way* some sort of technician or superior cook.

The caterer dietitian

The experiences of widespread food shortages such as occurred in Great Britain in the two world wars, if they achieved nothing else, have proved both the need and value of caterers with dietetic training in all large institutions. Before the 1939–45 war some 'public' schools had already appointed a dietitian-caterer, and found that not only were the pupils better fed, but also that they were spending less money on food. In state schools factories and other big employers, canteen caterers with dietetic training are needed.

The training of such people should be similar to that of the therapeutic dietitian, with the addition of large-scale catering and institutional management. They must be directly responsible in their professional appointments to the head of the institution and work in close co-operation with any medical officer appointed to oversee the health of those working in the institution. If, as in many long-stay hospitals and other residential communities, there is a garden or farm producing food for the residents, the caterer-dietitian should be able to advise on what should be grown.

The public health dietitian

This career overlaps with the previous one, but the scope of the work is considerably wider. Every area health authority and local authority needs the services of fully trained dietitians. The duties of such a person may be very varied and demand initiative, foresight and scientific insight, together with a capacity for handling people. Diet surveys need to be made in the home and in public institutions, especially in times of economic stress when spending may be restricted. Experiments in food consumption in community or school may be required, and advice and education in healthy dietary habits in schools, clinics, sports and recreational centres should always be available from the dietitian. The local authority dietitian should be expected to report on the chemical nature of the food served in school canteens, on its vitamin, protein and energy content. Dietitians are also needed in social service and social security departments, to advise on the nutritional state of their clients and the adequate level of financial help for those in need. (I have a clear memory of the great storm of interest that broke over our home when, in 1933, the British Medical Association first attempted, in defiance of the government of the day, to assess the minimal weekly cost of an adequate diet.)

While the hospital dietitian's work is at best curative, but mainly palliative, that of the caterer and public health dietitian is both preventive and economic. So far the hospitals have attracted the greater number of dietitians, because the career prospects were obvious and the emotional appeal the strongest, for it must be confessed that the cures produced by dietary treatment give the dietitian a source of drama and power. This is totally lacking in the day-by-day practice of preventive dietetics which, like all aspects of preventive medicine, has relatively lacked governmental support. However, now and in the future, in both developed and developing countries, just as in medicine, the spearpoint of effective progress is in preventive and educational dietetics. It is to be hoped that the openings in the future for applying the advancing knowledge in human nutrition will be found at all levels in the public services. It will be far more cost-effective to the tax- and rate-payer to reduce, by sound dietary advice and management, the incidence of tooth decay or diabetes than it is to treat the ravages of these diseases as they develop in our population.

In all these areas, then, the work is both scientific and practical, and needs a thorough training in scientific method, including research method. This division into three parts is, of course, arbitrary, and any one person may find herself moving from one to another area of work at different times. The common qualifications needed for such a person are a university degree course, including the fundamental sciences of chemistry, physiology and nutrition, practical studies in catering and dietetics, but also knowledge of management and personal relationships. It is to be hoped that a 4-year degree course (or a 3-year course followed by a single year's intensive practical training) can provide both the fundamental and applied knowledge in these fields, and the practical experience needed, together with an insight into the investigative approach to some of the work of the public health dietitian.

Be your own dietitian

Since many of the principles of nutrition (upon which sound dietetics is based), are essentially very simple, they can be readily understood by any person who has followed school courses in chemistry and biology up to the age of 16. These people could, by intelligently applying what they have learned by reading a book like this one, or from following a school course in home economics, become their own dietitian, so far as catering for themselves and their healthy familes are concerned. The hospital, catering and public service dietitians provide the specialist backing up service where a family-based do-it-yourself approach is no longer possible. It is, however, in the dietitian-at-home, you and me feeding ourselves, that most of the practice of dietetic knowledge will be applied, and a reasonable provision of knowledge in the whole population should parallel the special training of the professional dietitian.

2

Fundamentals of dietetics

Food may be defined as any substance which, when taken into the living organism enables it to grow and to maintain its health. For animals, this includes all solid foods, water and substances dissolved in water that enter the gastro-intestinal tract (gut) by the mouth. It excludes the flavouring materials that make food interesting, though these must be considered because, by stimulating the appetite, they favour the ingestion of the foodstuffs of major importance. Food need not enter the body by the gut, for it can be introduced directly into the circulation as, for example, a 5% glucose in water solution. The oxygen extracted from the air by the lungs is *not* regarded as a food, nor are drugs etc, even when they are given by mouth or by injection to supplement naturally occurring foodstuffs or substances formed in the body. As in all such definitions there is nothing clear-cut about the limits of the definition of what is a food. We will have to let the subject rest there.

In growth an organism adds to its substance, and the additions must come from outside, i.e. from its food, for it cannot create new matter out of nothing as this would be contrary to all scientific expectation. Food is needed also for maintenance of the living body. A living being exists solely by maintaining a state of imbalance between itself and its surroundings and to maintain this state it needs a constant supply of energy. It also continually loses some of its substance and this loss must be continually made good from the foodstuffs eaten.

The ways in which food enables the body to grow or to maintain itself are threefold:
(1) It supplies material for the production of energy (see Chapter 6).
(2) It supplies material for the building and repair of tissues (see Chapter 8).
(3) It supplies materials that, often in very small amounts, control and regulate the growth, repair and energy providing aspects of daily life (see Chapters 9 and 10).

Energy production

Energy is produced from foods almost entirely as a result of oxidation of their constituent carbohydrates, fats and proteins. Within the cells of the body, oxygen, coming originally from the air we breathe, is caused to react with substances derived from foods in a carefully controlled manner, so that as much as possible of the energy released in the oxidation reactions is trapped in a form that the cells can use for other functions. Some of the energy released in oxidation reactions appears immediately as heat and the great majority of other energy-needing functions convert the energy trapped in the oxidation process ultimately into heat. Some will be retained or expressed as physical or chemical work. Energy is measured in terms of *Joules* (see Chapter 5, page 32) and the energy content of a food is spoken of as the number of joules a weighed amount (usually 100 grams) will produce when it is oxidised.

Building and repair materials

These are mainly of three kinds: proteins, some fats and some inorganic materials. All the living cells of the body contain many kinds of protein. Most are present as *enzymes* which act as *catalysts*, enabling the living cells to carry out their many chemical reactions which could not occur without the protein enzymes. When cells grow or new cells are formed, more protein is needed. This has to be supplied from the food. When cells die and are broken down, although some of the protein can be re-used, some is lost to the body and again this must be replaced by food protein. All cell walls are made of a fatty substance which contains polyunsaturated fatty acids (see page 52). Since these are not made in the human body, they must be provided in the food when new cells are being made. Nerve tissue contains a great deal of cell-wall material so an adequate supply of this special fat must be available when the brain is growing (before birth and for the first two years of life thereafter).

The supporting skeleton needs a continual supply of calcium in the food, and the blood a supply of iron. Both these metallic substances are lost in normal daily life and the losses must be made up from the food. These subjects will be covered in detail in Chapter 9.

Controlling and regulating materials

In addition to sugars, fats, proteins and the inorganic substances mentioned in the preceding paragraphs, the body needs the materials that enable cellular oxidation to proceed in an ordinary and regulatable manner, or which help the body to lay down tissues in an orderly fashion. These substances need to be present only in minute amounts. The chemist calls them catalysts. The biochemist finds many of them acting as *co-enzymes* or carriers, enabling the protein enzymes to do their jobs in cells. Physiologists recognise others, which can be made in the body, as *hormones*. When they are composed of organic compounds which cannot be made in the body but must be found, preformed, in the food, they receive the name *vitamin*. Some inorganic substances, e.g. iron, calcium and copper act in the body as co-enzymes. One, iodine, is a part of the hormone *thyroxine*. These materials are described fully in Chapters 9 and 10.

The study of nutrition, then, is based upon energy, proteins, inorganic materials and the vitamins, when we treat it from a physical and chemical standpoint. It is based upon energy transformation, body building, and the regulation of these processes, when we consider it from the physiological viewpoint. Chemistry and physics deal with what things *are*, but physiology and biochemistry with what they *do*, i.e. what are their functions. As said above, fats, carbohydrates and (to a lesser extent) proteins, provide energy. Proteins, some fats and some inorganic materials are used for building processes. Inorganic materials and vitamins catalyse and regulate both energy transformation and body building.

At this point I must emphasise that foods (except a very few man-made substances) contain the different chemical and physiological classes of substances described above in different amounts and combinations. *No one food provides all the substances needed in a diet*, and very few even approximate to this ideal. It would be well at this point to give the analysis of some ordinary foods and show how all are lacking in one or more of the necessary components of an adequate diet. I have chosen bread, milk, meat and potatoes and have used tables from *The Composition of Foods* (McCance & Widdowson, 1967). The results are displayed in Table 2.1. Each column represents one of nine important nutritional components of foodstuffs, and each line shows the amount of each component present in 100 grams of the food. I should say here that throughout this book I will always refer to 100 grams of a food (whether solid or liquid) when describing its composition. This weight is about $3\frac{1}{2}$ ounces and will therefore be more easily 'recognised' in practice than the S.I. standard mass of 1 kilogram. You will see that beef steak tops the list for fat and protein per 100g eaten, bread for carbohydrates, while milk is much the best for calcium, meat for iron, milk for vitamin A, bread for vitamin B and potatoes for vitamin C. Potatoes have no fat and very little protein, whereas meat has no carbohydrate. Beef and potatotes have little calcium, while milk has little iron. Bread and potatoes have no vitamin A, and meat no vitamin C, while milk contains it in small amounts.

Table 2.1 Nutritional components provided by 100 grams of basic foods.

Food	Protein g	Fat g	Available CHO g	Energy kJ	Calcium mg	Iron mg	Vitamins A mg	B mg	C mg
White bread	8.1	1.4	51.8	1030	92.0	1.83	0	0.63	nil
Beef steak	19.4	10.6	nil	735	5.3	4.30	trace	0.25	nil
Fresh milk (whole)	3.2	3.9	4.9	280	120.0	0.07	100–150	0.14	7.0
Potatoes (stored)	2.1	trace	20.8	368	7.7	0.74	trace	0.39	8–30

This little example brings out at once one of the fundamental principles of dietetics. *Only a mixed diet can give us the essential energy, protein, inorganic materials and vitamins*. When, as will be apparent later on, we have considered all the necessary items of a good diet in detail, a mixture of these four foods, which form a large part of the diet of most people, will be seen to be inadequate to maintain the best state of health. A much more varied diet is required. One important function of dietetics is to discover what is the best diet. The deficits in one food, e.g. vitamin C in bread, must be made up by other foods which add the missing ingredient(s). The term *balanced diet* has been used to describe one with no deficit, though perhaps the alternative term, *optimal diet*, is preferable. This term implies that the diet is so well conceived that it cannot be improved by the addition to it of any foodstuff. The dietitian must always aim at and direct people to an optimal diet. It must be made clear that *there is no one optimal diet*, but an *indefinite number of ways of obtaining an optimal diet*. Although a reasonable excess of most constituents never does anyone any harm, any excess in terms of joules or energy *may* be deposited as fat, and gross excess of some substances may be harmful. Deficits of any component are, *in the long run*, severely harmful. With many deficits the body may manage to survive for some months or even years (as was seen in Europe in the 1939–45 war, and is to be seen nowadays in many parts of the world), but these deficits display themselves in the general lassitude of such peoples, their liability to develop anaemia and infectious diseases and their death rates, maternal and infantile mortality rates.

The body is, however, extremely adaptable, thus custom and habit can provide a great range of optimal diets from the almost entirely meat-eating habit of the Eskimo to the almost entirely herbivorous Hindu and Kikuyu. It has been found that in temperate climates people can live for a year on a diet consisting exclusively of meat, fish and eggs, while we also have the vegetarians, living on cheese, eggs, milk, nuts, fruits and vegetables who are, both physically and mentally, as good as, *but not better than*, the rest of us. Vegans, who eliminate all animal products from the diet, including milk products and eggs, may run short of one of the B vitamins and develop pernicious anaemia as a result.

Twenty years ago, so far as the science of nutrition was concerned, it was confidently stated that the United States of America was the best-fed nation. This was ascribed to the prosperity of that country and the development of nutrition as a science at the beginning of the twentieth century. Canada, Australia, New Zealand and the 'white' races of Southern Africa approached the same level, as did the Scandinavian countries. Britain, as a result of the 1939–45 war, greatly improved its standards and by 1955, at the end of food rationing and with increasing prosperity, was heading towards the American standards. Even before the war, food intakes and growth patterns of *middle-class* English children were as good as those of the Americans, while statistics obtained by the London County Council in 1959 showed improvements over 1949 in the growth of children from state schools.

The situation in West Germany, the Benelux Countries, Switzerland and France is similar, but Eastern Europe and the Mediterranean Countries are less well fed. The diets of the great masses of people in Southern America, Africa and Asia (though we do not know very much about China, and Japan approaches the North American standard) are sufficient only to maintain life. Thus the expectation of life in India is only half of that in Great Britain and undernourishment must play a part in this reduction. Much of the incidence of tuberculosis, other infections and some of the maternal and infant mortality are due to inadequate food. Two-thirds of the world's population, by the standards of nutritional scientists, get too little energy in their foods and the deficit in proteins, inorganic materials and vitamins is probably greater still.

However, in North America and Western Europe there is now some evidence that we are over-eating and the consequences of obesity, together with arterial disease and diabetes (both perhaps due to too much of the 'wrong' foods) are needlessly shortening life expectation in these countries.

Whether it is undernourishment or malnutrition that shortens life, the science of nutrition, correctly applied, will promote good health and an active and long life which are the birthright of us all. Both national, e.g. the British wartime Ministry of Food, and international organisations, e.g. the Food and Agriculture Organisation (FAO) of the United Nations, attempt this application of knowledge, though their efforts are frequently frustrated by local customs or economic conditions. Some people doubt whether the world, with its physical resources and energy available, can ever hope to feed its present or future population to an adequate level for an indefinite future. The nutritional scientist should consider not only what is desirable, but look at the practical implications for the world of an attempt to achieve this goal of worldwide nutritional adequacy.

It has been shown that in the better-fed nations the intake of energy-providing and body-building foods are satisfactory, but that the intake of foods providing inorganic materials and vitamins could be improved. We will set out here a preliminary tabular statement showing what foodstuffs are valuable for which purpose, and how they are obtained (Table 2.2.).

Table 2.2

Purpose of food	Chemical nature	Source
Energy production	Fats, starches, sugars and proteins	Dripping, lard, suet, butter, margarine, vegetable oils, cheese, bacon, cereals, sugar, dried fruits, nuts, pulses and potatoes.
Building and repair	Proteins, calcium and iron	Milk, cheese, eggs, meat, fish, cereals and pulses
Control and regulation	Calcium, iron iodine, phosphorus, the vitamins	Milk, cheese, eggs, bacon, some fruit and vegetables and fatty fish

The three columns represent respectively the attitudes of the physiologist (dealing with bodily and nutritional function), the chemist and of the caterer. The nutritional scientist must, of course, keep all three simultaneously in mind. The above classification is not perfect, however, nor is the alignment between columns and rows the same in all countries. Although we in Great Britain obtain only about 10% of our energy from protein, the Eskimo perforce obtains 44% from protein. We obtain little of our protein from the pulses, but in some tropical countries beans, in one form or another, form a major source of protein. The inorganic materials in the food are needed, mainly in small amounts, for control and regulation, but calcium and phosphorus, in addition to their catalytic functions, are required in relatively enormous amounts for skeletal growth and maintenance, with the result that *the child's and the adolescent's need for calcium is much greater than the adult's*. Further, while it is true that we get our energy-containing foods mainly from the grocer and the baker, and our body-building foods from the dairyman, butcher and fishmonger, we cannot say that we get the substances for control and regulation from the greengrocer. Thus calcium comes in large amounts from milk and cheese, iron from eggs and liver, and vitamin D (just to take one example) from eggs, milk and the fat fish. Among fruits the grape, apple and pear are worthless for all vitamins, as is the marrow among vegetables. For the purpose of supplying vitamin C, sometimes in short supply in many institutions owing to large losses in bulk catering methods, the composition of fruit and vegetables must be closely scrutinised using the appropriate tables.

The special places of cheese and bacon should be considered. Both supply up to 1.8 MJ/100g of energy, cheese is 20–30% protein and bacon is 7–14% protein and while bacon is a rich source of thiamine, cheese supplies calcium, vitamin A and riboflavine. Thus both belong in all three lines of Table 2.2. A similar position is held by herrings, but the very success of the promotion of consumption of herrings, kippers and bloaters has resulted in a grave reduction of this most valuable food from the waters around Great Britain. Its cost in the shops is in 1977 five times what it was 6 years ago. In 1971 it was the cheapest energy source (along with Cheddar cheese), 100g supplied 0.8 MJ, and contained 17g of protein. Herrings were also a good source of calcium, iodine, vitamins A and D and nicotinic acid. Milk is of course comparable to cheese, but in a dilute watery form. A litre of milk contains the solid matter of 50–80g of cheese.

These foods are mentioned for three reasons:

(1) To show that generalisations about, and tabular arrangements of foods for energy, building or control have their drawbacks and pitfalls.
(2) To bring out the erratic distribution of vitamins among foods.
(3) To emphasise the great value of bacon, cheese, milk and herrings in dietetics.

As has already been mentioned, the foods deficient in the diets of even the best-fed countries are the ones that supply inorganic materials and vitamins. These are the dairy products, market garden products, i.e. green vegetables and summer fruits and fatty fish. It has been estimated that to obtain sufficient of these in the diet of Great Britain, an *increase* in production of 60–100% is required. Our soil and climate are probably unequalled for dairy, fruit and vegetable production and the requirement could easily be met. Our fish stocks, particularly of herrings, need the most careful control and management to ensure that the optimal amount is available for direct human consumption. To convert fish to animal feedingstuffs is a nutritional disaster.

3
The chemistry of carbohydrates, fats and proteins

Carbohydrates

These are a group of compounds of the elements carbon, hydrogen and oxygen. The latter two are present in the same proportion, two atoms of hydrogen to one of oxygen, as in water, hence the name carbohydrate, for *hudor* is the Greek for water. Carbohydrates are found in food either as *sugars* or as *starches* and *glycogen*. These latter materials are long straight or branched chains of many sugar molecules joined together. The chemical nature of the sugars determines their properties, their function in living tissues and how starches are formed and broken down, so this chemical nature will now be described.

Monosaccharides

These are the simplest sugars known to the chemist and physiologist. They may consist of 4 or 5, but usually of 6 carbon atoms, the same number of oxygen atoms and twice the number of hydrogen atoms. Usually sugar molecules exist in a ring form, the ring containing all but one of the carbons and an oxygen atom. The remaining carbon, the hydrogen and the other oxygen atoms are placed 'above' or 'below' the ring. Glucose is a simple sugar, containing in each molecule 6 carbon, 12 hydrogen and 6 oxygen atoms. Thus it has an empirical formula $C_6H_{12}O_6$. An attempt to draw its three-dimensional molecular structure on a two-dimensional flat surface is shown in Fig. 3.1. Fructose and galactose are the other two monosaccharides of major nutritional importance. They too have the same empirical formula as glucose, but differ, as is seen in Fig. 3.1, in the disposition of the accessory atoms and groups around the basic carbon and oxygen ring structure. These structural differences are of great importance once the monosaccharides enter the living body, for they determine the ways in which they can be used. These three ways of arranging the same carbon, hydrogen and oxygen atoms around the basic ring structure are not the only possible arrangements. Many other configurations are possible, and some exist in various plant and bacterial carbohydrates.

The monosaccharides readily combine into pairs, known as *disaccharides*. Those of importance in nutrition are *sucrose*, formed from one molecule of glucose and one of fructose, *lactose*, formed from glucose and galactose, and *maltose*, formed from two glucose molecules. In each case a molecule of

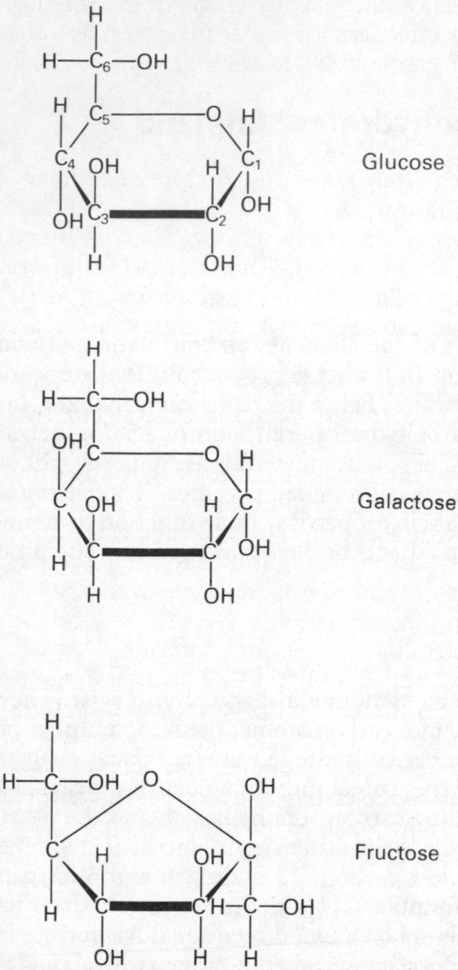

Fig. 3.1 Structural formulae for glucose, galactose and fructose.

water is lost when the two monosaccharides thus combine, so the empirical fomulae of disaccharide molecules is $C_{12}H_{22}O_{11}$.

Sugars and polarised light

Light beams behave as though the rays are vibrating transversely to the direction of the beam. Special optical apparatus produces rays all vibrating in the same plane, known as polarised light. Solutions of compounds with asymmetry in their structure rotate the plane of vibration of light passing through them. All three monosaccharides are asymmetrical at carbons 1 to 4. Glucose rotates the plane of polarisation in one direction, fructose more strongly in the opposite direction. In forming sucrose, the final compound rotates light in the same direction as glucose. Breaking sucrose down to a mixture of glucose and sucrose thus results in an inversion of the rotation direction. Enzymes that cause this effect are known as invertases and the resultant mixture of glucose and fructose is called *invert sugar*.

Polysaccharides

These are chain molecules formed from many monosaccharides linked together. The chains can be straight or branched and can be formed from any of the 6-carbon monosaccharides already described, from 5-carbon sugars, or from the *amino sugars*, related compounds having an $-NH_2$ group in place of one of the $-OH$ groups. The only polysaccharides of major nutritional importance, because they can be digested in the human gut, are *starches* and *glycogen*.

Starches and glycogen are formed from chains of glucose molecules. *Amylose* is a straight-chain form of starch, containing several hundred glucose molecules, linked 'head for tail' between carbon 1 of one glucose molecule and carbon 4 of the next (as in maltose, a molecule of water is lost in forming the link). *Amylopectin* and glycogen are branched chains. In these, a second link is formed, between carbon 6 of one unit and carbon 1 of another. These branches occur at 18–20 glucose unit intervals in glycogen, but at longer intervals in amylopectin. Many thousand glucose units may be present in a single branched chain polysaccharide.

Many other polysaccharides exist. *Cellulose*, present in all plant cell walls, is formed, like starch, from glucose, but the link is different and we cannot digest it. *Inulin* is a polysaccharide formed from fructose, and *agar* from galactose. These two polysaccharides are found in the daisy family of flowering plants and in seaweeds respectively. Both, like amino sugar polysaccharides and polysaccharides formed from pentoses by some plants, cannot be digested by man. The nutritional significance of these non-digestible materials will be described later (p. 133).

Occurrence of carbohydrates

Glucose appears to be the keystone of metabolism in both plants and animals. Thus it is the main product of photosynthesis in green plants, and, in starch, is their main storage material in many seed, root or stem storage organs. It is only rarely found free in plant material, grapes being the most significant exception. It is present in human blood, at about 80–120 mg/100 ml blood (5–6 mmol/litre), and is the only sugar that plays a major role in human metabolism. Glycogen is found in the liver and muscles of animals. Fructose is found free in some fruits, but galactose occurs only in combination, as lactose in milk.

Of the disaccharides, sucrose is widely distributed in plant fruits and other tissues. It is, in fact, the common 'sugar' of regular daily use, our nutritional supplies coming from sugar cane and sugar beet. Maltose is formed from the starch of grain seeds when these begin to germinate.

The *sweetness* of sugars lies principally in the fructose molecule. This is twice as sweet, molecule for molecule, as is sucrose, three times sweeter than glucose and eight times as sweet as lactose. Infants perhaps, then, do not acquire a 'sweet tooth' from mother's milk so much as from sucrose added to artificial feeds.

Fats

The fats are compounds of *glycerol* with *fatty acids*. Glycerol (also known commercially as *glycerine*), which is not unlike a 3-carbon sugar in structure is commonly depicted as follows:

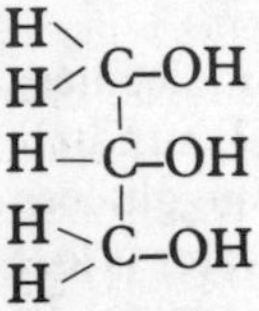

$$
\begin{array}{l}
\text{H} \diagdown \\
\text{H} \diagup \text{C--OH} \\
\text{H--C--OH} \quad \text{or } CH_2OH.CH\ OH.CH_2OH \\
\text{H} \diagdown \text{C--OH} \\
\text{H} \diagup
\end{array}
$$

The fatty acids consist of chains of carbon and hydrogen atoms terminating at one end in the following acidic group $-\underset{\underset{O}{\|}}{C}-OH$. Butyric acid is thus

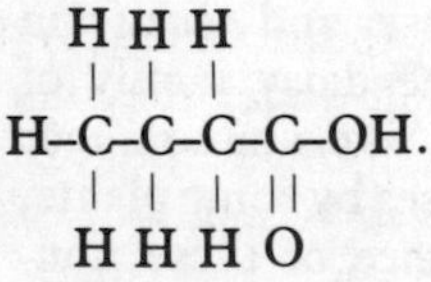

$$
\begin{array}{l}
\text{H H H} \\
\,\,|\,\,\,|\,\,\,| \\
\text{H--C--C--C--C--OH.} \\
\,\,\,|\,\,\,\,|\,\,\,\,|\,\,\,\,\| \\
\,\,\,\text{H H H O}
\end{array}
$$

This formula is often abbreviated to $C_3H_7.COOH$. Sometimes there are double bonds between adjacent carbon atoms, with the loss of two hydrogen atoms:

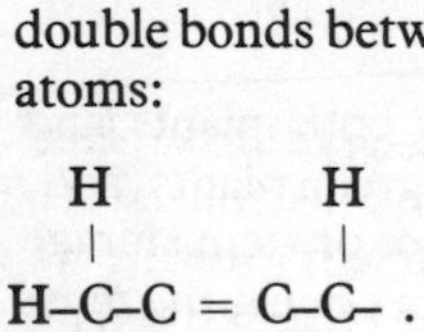

$$
\begin{array}{l}
\text{H} \qquad\quad \text{H} \\
\,|\qquad\quad\,| \\
\text{H--C--C} = \text{C--C--} . \\
\,\,|\,\,\,|\qquad|\,\,\,| \\
\,\,\text{H H}\quad\text{H H}
\end{array}
$$

Many fatty acids exist with 16, 18 or 20 carbon atoms in the chain. Thus *stearic* acid contains 18 carbons, and no double bonds, *oleic* acid also contains 18 carbons, with one double bond, *palmitic* acid has 16 carbons, and linoleic acid has 18, with two double bonds. Oleic and linoleic acids are known as *unsaturated* fatty acids, for they can accept additional hydrogen at the sites of the double bonds. Stearic acid is often written as $C_{17}H_{35}.COOH$ and oleic acid as $C_{17}H_{33}.COOH$.

When a fatty acid combines with glycerol a water molecule is lost, thus:

$CH_2OH.CHOH.CH_2O \overline{[H + HO]} OC.C_3H_7 \rightarrow$

$CH_2OH.CHOH.CH_2O.OC.C_3H_7$ (glyceryl monobutyrate)
The dotted line indicating the water molecule lost.

Rarely in a complete fat is only one fatty acid present. Usually three different fatty acids are found attached to the glycerol molecule: thus in butter the main fat is glyceryl butyro-oleostearate, one molecule of each of the three acids being combined with the glycerol molecule. The final nature of a fat or oil substance, whether it be hard like lamb dripping, soft like beef dripping or butter, or liquid, like fish or vegetable oils, is determined by the fatty acids that are present in the fat.

Spontaneous chemical changes can take place in a fat. In the presence of water and some micro-organisms, the links between glycerol and the fatty acids can be split. The free acids may give an unpleasant taste, as when butter becomes rancid. Another change results from oxidation reactions at the site of the double bonds in the unsaturated fatty acids. Such reactions may, if uncontrolled, produce peroxide groupings which can have far-reaching and harmful effects upon living tissues.

Occurrence of fats

All living cells contain traces of fat in their structure, for fatty acids are among the components of cell wall and other intracellular membrane structures. In mammals and birds, fat deposits and stores are found throughout the body: between muscles, around internal organs and under the skin. Many fish have fat stored exclusively in the liver, but in the herring, for example, it is present throughout the flesh. In the vegetable kingdom, fats are found in the fruiting bodies of various plants, such as olives, maize, palm nuts, to name but a few.

Proteins

The word *protein* is derived from Greek, and means 'holding the first place'. Proteins literally hold the first place in the architecture and machinery of all living things. Without them no life can exist. No plant can grow or trap sunlight, no baby can be born or reared unless proteins have been made. There is an enormous range of proteins, plant proteins, animal proteins, human proteins—millions of them, all different—but all built up from the same 20 building blocks, the amino acids, in long chains. These can be arranged in any order and there may be several hundred amino acids in a single protein molecule. You can readily see how many proteins can be made when you think that there are 20 possible different amino acids in the first place of the chain, 20 in the second, 20 in the third and so on for 400 places. The number is $20 \times 20 \times 20$, perhaps 400 times. The number is unimaginably huge—there are over three million different ways of arranging amino acids in the first 5 places alone! The amino acids themselves are relatively simple substances. If we start with acetic acid, the acid of vinegar, we can write its structural formula thus:

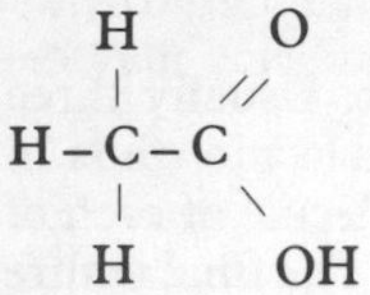

$$\begin{array}{ccc} H & O & \\ | & // & \\ H - C - C & & \text{or } CH_3.COOH \\ | & \backslash & \\ H & OH & \end{array}$$

which you will recognise is the simplest of the fatty acid series.

To make an amino acid we replace a hydrogen atom, on the carbon *next to the one* with the =O on it, with an amino group, –NH₂ (which is very closely related to ammonia, NH₃). Aminoacetic acid, also known as *glycine*, is thus:

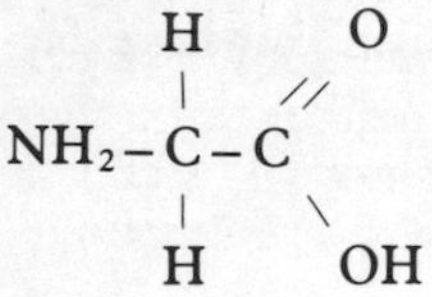

$$\begin{array}{ccc} H & O & \\ | & // & \\ NH_2 - C - C & & \text{or } CH_2NH_2.COOH \\ | & \backslash & \\ H & OH & \end{array}$$

Proprionic acid is the next fatty acid up the series from acetic acid. Its formula is $CH_3.CH_2.COOH$. The corresponding amino acid, *alamine* has the following structure:

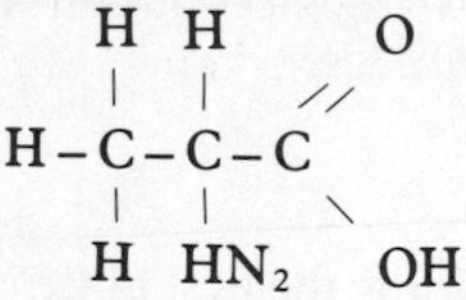

$$\begin{array}{cccc} H & H & O & \\ | & | & // & \\ H - C - C - C & & \text{or } CH_3CH\ NH_2.COOH \\ | & | & \backslash & \\ H & HN_2 & OH & \end{array}$$

The carbon atom with the –NH₂ group attached, known as the a-carbon and having *four different* chemical groups attached to it, may exist with them in two different spatial arrangements, which are the mirror-image of each other. *All* amino acids in proteins exist in one of these arrangements only, the mirror images never being found naturally, though chemists can make them artificially.

The other amino acids will differ from alamine and glycine at the left hand end of the molecules as they are shown above. The bit –CH NH₂.COOH is common to all of them. In glycine a hydrogen is added, in alamine CH₃ is added, and in the others various short chains or rings of carbon atoms, with hydrogen, oxygen, sulphur or even further NH₂ groups also present. This end of the molecule is frequently given the single letter 'R', so the general formula for amino acids is R.CH NH_2.COOH.

When amino acids combine to form proteins, they do this through the NH_2 group of one amino acid reacting with the OH of another amino acid, splitting of water, H.OH, in the process. A chain of amino acids may be written as:

$$
\begin{array}{cccccc}
R & H & O & R & H & O \\
| & | \ \ H & || & | & | & || \\
C & N \ \ | \ \ C & C & N & C & \\
| \ \ C & C & N \ \ | \ \ C & C & N & \cdots \cdots \\
H \ || & | & | \ \ H & || & | & | \\
O & R & H & O & R & H
\end{array}
$$

When the whole thing is put together in three dimensions, the R side-chains have to fit together without colliding with each other. Side-chains consisting only of carbon and hydrogen tend to come together, for they shun water. Side-chains with oxygen or NH_2 groups will mix with water so these also occupy adjacent places when the peptide chain of a protein folds itself up, as it always will if it can.

Side chains of some amino acids can be made in the body, but those of 9 amino acids must be present in the diet, as must the NH_2 groups themselves. The nine essential acids are histidine, isoleucine, leucine, lysine, methionine, phenylalanine, threonine, tryptophan and valine. Histidine is needed in children only.

Now that this simple description of the chemical nature of the three chief components of food has been given, Chapters 5 and 7 will consider them in relation to energy production (carbohydrates and fats principally) and body growth (proteins).

4
Digestion, absorption and metabolism of food

An understanding of what happens to foods after they are eaten to the time when they reappear in the outside world as carbon dioxide, water and simple nitrogenous compounds, is essential to the understanding of nutrition and practical problems in dietetics. The following chapter is but the briefest sketch, and though perhaps enough for practical purposes is by no means the whole truth.

Digestion

Most of the foods which we eat are insoluble in water. The body is at least 60% water, and the tissues where the chemical activities subserving life take place are at least 70% water, and it is in this water that those activities occur. Consequently food must be rendered *soluble*. Solubility is not enough. Egg-white proteins are dissolved in water, but they will not pass through animal membranes. Their molecules are too large. So they cannot diffuse through the walls of the small intestine into the blood stream. They must therefore be made *diffusible*. But even diffusibility is not enough. Cane sugar is diffusible through animal membranes. None the less cane sugar, if it gets into the blood stream, is of no use to the body. It is excreted at once in the urine. Each substance in food has to become usable by the body cells—call it *metabolisable*.

To render foods soluble, diffusible and metabolisable the body uses the alimentary tract, a set of tubular organs passing from mouth to anus, a part of the external world tucked into and through the body, some 6.5 m long in the dead body, but in life, such is its tone and elasticity, only 2.7 m in length. The functions of this tract are partly mechanical and partly chemical—the food has to be broken up physically into smaller and smaller pieces, and also, chemically, into simpler and simpler compounds. To bring about the physical changes there is the grinding apparatus of the teeth, but further along the tract there are the movements, such as peristalsis, which produce maceration of the food. The physical grinding and maceration, plus the chemical changes brought about in the tract we term digestion.

The term indigestion
Indigestion has two different meanings. The physiologist means by *indigestible* a food substance which the enzymes in the alimentary tract have difficulty in changing to simpler substances, and which the small intestine has difficulty in absorbing. In other words, when eaten it is apt to appear at

the distant end of the alimentary tract unchanged in part or *in toto*. Medicinal paraffin oil is an example; cellulose and phytates are others. We have no enzymes for cellulose and plant cell wall substances in the alimentary tract, but we have bacteria which attack them and produce gases—carbon dioxide, methane and hydrogen—which distend the colon and cause pain. In youth and middle age the gut walls can pass much of this gas into the blood stream, but they lose this power later in life. So salads and fruits such as apples may double up the elderly with wind.

Indigestion to the physician means pain arising from the alimentary tract consequent on taking food. But it should be realised that the food may be digestible in the physiological sense and yet cause indigestion. It very often is true that indigestion follows the taking of indigestible substances, but not necessarily so. Over-activity of the muscles of the walls of the stomach and over-secretion of acid is accompanied by pain, and the fault lies not with the food eaten but with the irritability of the nervous system of the eater. This is a point worth stressing in view of the habit of nervous folk of cutting out this or that food from their diets because the eating of it has been followed by pain.

Digestive Enzymes

To produce complete chemical digestion of foodstuffs the alimentary tract produces a whole battery of enzymes. Generic terms for the enzymes end in 'ase'—protease for protein splitting, lipase for fat splitting, amylase for starch splitting, sucrase for cane sugar splitting enzymes, and so on. Often an enzyme will be given a specific name—as it were a Christian name—e.g. the protease of the gastric juice is called pepsin.

The huge chains of amino acids which are proteins have points of attack for different proteases. Thus pepsin will attack at one type of linkage, and trypsin and chymotrypsin (proteases made by the pancreas) will attack at others. Even when these have done their worst, or rather best, there are still other peptidases, to complete the work of digesting the proteins to amino acids, and only in this form are they useful to the body. No such complication is necessary with fats and the lipase. Fats are relatively uncomplicated substances. There may be a lipase in the stomach juices in infants, but the main lipase is that of the pancreatic juice which splits fats to fatty acid and glycerol (see p. 26).

Carbohydrates, on the other hand, can be very complicated, though their individual building stones are few (glucose mainly). There is an amylase, called ptyalin, in saliva and another, called amylopsin, in the pancreatic juice, which work upon cooked starch and change it to maltose (pp. 22 and 26). Maltose is useless to the body unless digested to glucose by the maltase of the cells lining the small intestine. Similarly sucrose (or cane sugar) must be digested to glucose and fructose by sucrase, and lactose (milk sugar) to glucose and galactose by lactase.

It is doubtful if the human alimentary tract can digest uncooked starch. It probably passes unchanged into the large intestine, where it meets bacteria which turn it into 'wind'.

Digestion in the mouth

The chief function of the mouth is the breaking up of the food into small pieces convenient to swallow. This is done by the combined action of teeth and tongue. Thorough chewing of food is important, and many cases of dyspepsia are produced and continued by imperfections of teeth and dentures. At the same time that food is chewed it is mixed with the slimy secretion of the 3 main pairs of salivary glands and other scattered glands. The sliminess is due to mucin, a curious substance compounded of carbohydrate and protein. Its function is to make food slippery. In addition, any cooked starch in the food eaten is digested to dextrins and maltose by the salivary amylase. Though this enzyme is accidental (most animals have it, though in a state of nature they do not meet cooked starch) it is as well to take advantage of it. Porous foods, such as rusks, are easily penetrable by saliva (whereas new bread is not), and therefore are easily digestible by ptyalin.

The volume of saliva varies with the condition of the body, the nature and tastiness of the food. A thirsty person cannot produce saliva, which should be remembered in feeding a dehydrated patient. Wet foods evoke less saliva than dry foods, but the most potent factor in producing saliva is the taste or smell of the food. Acidity always evokes salivation, possibly to neutralise the acid. Slight astringency does the same. And if the food is liked or the person hungry the flow of saliva is greatest. (This is true, too, of gastric juice.)

One other function of saliva is in keeping the mouth clean. Fever suppresses salivation and the mouth gets foul. All these facts about saliva are worth remembering in practical dietetics.

The food when chewed passes down the oesophagus (which has no functions other than being a connecting tube) to the stomach. Here it is retained from one to five hours, or even longer.

Digestion in the stomach

The stomach acts as (1) a reservoir, (2) a macerating organ, (3) a steriliser, (4) a temperature regulator, (5) a digester of proteins, and (6) a secreter of the substance ('intrinsic factor') connected with the absorption of vitamin B_{12} from the intestine.

The stomach as a reservoir

The practical convenience of having a reservoir early in the alimentary tract is obvious. Its capacity determines the frequency with which a person has to eat. The stomach's capacity (which varies very much from person to person) is, generally speaking, not enough for the one-meal-a-day man, though workers in the Johannesburg gold mines use that practice! Modern work seems to indicate that despite man's possessing a stomach reservoir, 'little and often' is the best rule in taking meals.

The stomach as a macerating organ

Maceration takes place partly due to the secretion of gastric juice and partly to movements of the stomach wall. The secretion of gastric juice depends upon two factors: (1) a nervous reflex starting from nerve organs in the tongue and nose, (2) the production in the walls of the stomach of two hormones which excite the secretory cells of the glands of the stomach to secrete.

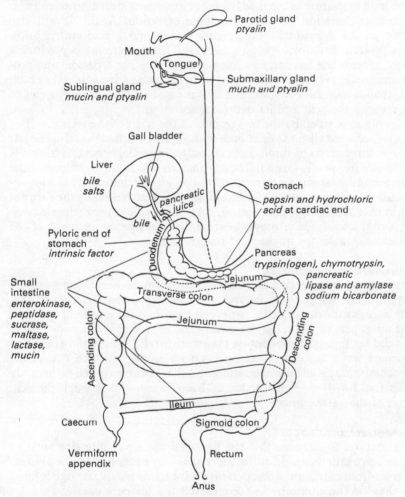

Fig. 4.1 The anatomy of the digestive tract.

The nervous reflex acts almost as soon as food is eaten (i.e. it begins within five minutes) and will continue for an hour to an hour and a half. With most people the more the food (and its setting) is liked, the greater the flow of gastric juice, and therefore, presumably, the better the digestion.

Some foods directly (e.g. meat extracts and soups made from meat), and other foods when partially digested, set free from the walls of the stomach into the blood stream a hormone called gastrin, which further stimulates the cells to activity. The 'nervously' controlled juice is acid and contains pepsin; the 'chemically' evoked juice is acid but poor in pepsin.

The total secretion of gastric juice depends (*a*) on the nervous ('psychic') flow, whether brisk or sluggish, and (*b*) on the chemical flow, which depends on the nature of the food, whether it contains meat extracts, etc., or whether its digestion products stimulate secretion. Again, it will also depend on the individual. Some people secrete much acid gastric juice, others produce little or even no acid, and if either extreme is producing trouble appropriate feeding should be instituted. Thus a person who produces normally too much acid should avoid soups and foods he very much likes, should take milk and increase his fat consumption. (The proteins of milk take up the acid and fat depresses secretion.)

Maceration is aided by the movements of the walls of the stomach. The organ is U-shaped with the right limb of the U shorter than the left. The left limb remains quiescent throughout digestion; its walls behave as the walls of an elastic bag would do on filling it with material. In the right limb of the U annular indentations appear around the organ and these rings of contraction move slowly towards the far end of the stomach. Normally they are not deep in man, unless for some reason, such as organic disease, the stomach wall is overactive. These movements gently massage the contents of the stomach and make for mixing and maceration.

Sterilisation in the stomach

The concentration of hydrochloric acid in the stomach contents is usually great enough to kill putrefactive and many pathogenic bacteria, which may partly account for the fact that not everyone who drinks typhoid contaminated water gets typhoid. (At the time of the Boer War it was said that the Boers did not take typhoid because they were careful to eat before drinking suspicious water instead of taking it on an empty stomach.) Anyhow, hydrochloric acid is an antiseptic and stomach contents exposed to the air do not go foul for days. Acid-producing bacteria can slip through the acid barrier of the gastric juice.

Temperature regulation

It is natural to suppose that the lining of the small intestine with its intense corrugations would suffer more than any other part of the alimentary tract from extremes of temperature. Hot foods would damage it more than they do the stomach. In the stomach the temperatures of food are brought to normal body temperature. None the less, very hot foods are to be avoided—the incidence of cancer in the first parts of the alimentary tract among Chinese men, when it is almost absent among the women, who by convention take their meals after their husbands have finished indicates this. The limits of safety are said to be 7–54°C, though one has to admit that many people seem to be immune to going beyond such limits.

Digestion

The first stage of digestion of protein starts in the stomach. The hydrochloric acid unites with the protein, and the enzyme, pepsin, begins to digest it. It attacks the protein at vulnerable points in its structure, and thus produces simpler molecules, but even if digestion is prolonged these molecules are still quite large.

Secretion of the intrinsic factor for maturation of red blood corpuscles

For long it has been recognised that two factors are needed to ensure the maturation of red blood corpuscles, one coming from the food (called the extrinsic factor) and one from the lining of the stomach (the intrinsic factor). Now, it is established that the extrinsic factor is cobalamin or the vitamin B_{12}. This, by itself, injected into the blood stream can deal with pernicious anaemia and bring the blood picture back towards normal, and also the degeneration of the spinal cord seen in pernicious anaemia. Apparently the substance elaborated by the mucous membrane of the stomach is needed to transport the B_{12} across the mucous membrane of the small intestine (see p. 112).

Not much digestion of carbohydrates occurs in the stomach except perhaps at the quiet proximal arm of the U tube. Here, if starchy foods (e.g. puddings) are taken later in the meal, salivary digestion continues so long as the contents of that part of the stomach do not become markedly acid. None, however, of the digested products are absorbed from the stomach; nor is water, though if alcohol be taken with the meal some of that is absorbed.

Digestion in the small intestines

The contents of the stomach may begin to be pushed on into the duodenum within ten minutes after the meal is eaten, and from time to time material ('acid chyme') is passed on until the stomach is emptied. The time this takes varies with the individual and the amount and nature of the food. Fruits and lettuce get out remarkably quickly. Milk, eggs, gelatin and vegetables pass through quickly, while fish and meats take longer. Pork, contrary to belief, takes but little longer than lamb. Consequently the rate of passage of foods is not a measure of digestibility. What slows down the passage of foods is (a) the amount of acid they can absorb without becoming acid, (b) the amount of fat they contain, and (c) the difficulty with which they can be turned into smooth chyme. Nuts are notoriously slow—30 g of nuts will stay three hours in the stomach—and they are very compact, difficult to chew properly, and contain much fat.

The acid chyme passing into the duodenum is assailed by many digestive juices. The pancreas secretes trypsin, chymotrypsin (proteases), a lipase and an amylase in an alkaline medium; the liver and gall bladder pour out bile salts; the glands of the small intestine produce other proteases, and enterokinase, an enzyme which unmasks the proteolytic activity of trypsin and chymotrypsin.

The two trypsins tackle undigested proteins, and the ones acted on by pepsin, and convert them to polypeptides—linkages of four or more amino acids. These are digested by other peptidases, which attack the polypeptide chain at either end, to free amino acids and dipeptides.

The lipase digests the fat of the food to glycerol and fatty acids. This process is aided by the emulsifying action of bile salts and of the products of the lipolysis itself. It is not known how much of the triglyceride is broken down to free fatty acids or the intermediate compounds (mono- and diglycerides). Particles of unsplit fat, partially hydrolysed fat and free fatty acid can all be freely absorbed if the particle size is less than 0.5 micron. Both bile salts and pancreatic lipase are essential for fat digestion and absorption. After absorption, 50–60% of the fat is found, *as unsplit fat*, in the lymphatics. Much of this may have been reconstituted by the cells in the intestinal wall. This fat consists of the long-chain fatty acids. The remainder (principally short-chain fatty acid fats) passes to the liver in the portal blood.

The *amylase* attacks unchanged cooked starch and dextrins and changes them to maltose. It is also said to digest uncooked starch, but with difficulty. *Maltase* carries on the digestion of maltose to glucose. *Sucrase* converts cane sugar into glucose and fructose. *Lactase* changes lactose to glucose and galactose. These three disaccharidases are found principally within the cells lining the gut. The digestible carbohydrates of the food are now in the form in which they are metabolised.

Absorption of digestion products

Absorption in the small intestine

Practically all absorption of the products of digestion of food takes place in the *small intestine*, which is a remarkably efficient organ. Two-thirds of it can be removed in man without desperate interference with absorption; or it may be badly ulcerated, as in typhoid fever, and yet carry out absorption efficiently. For absorption to take place satisfactorily the foods must be in tiny particles so that they can be thoroughly digested; there must be bile salts present as well as digestive enzymes, and, of course, the intestines must be liberally supplied with blood and lymph. Four-fifths of the total water drunk is absorbed in the small intestine, and usually from 95 to 97% of the proteins, fats and carbohydrates eaten. If however the proteins are from vegetable foods less is absorbed, lentil proteins being particularly badly absorbed (80 per cent). If the fats have a high melting point less is absorbed, and sugars are more completely and rapidly digested and absorbed than starches. There is some difficulty in absorbing lactose as is described in the chapter on food allergies. Anything which hurries material along the small intestine—e.g. irritation due to bacteria, as in dysentery or due to purgatives—will hinder absorption, and undigested and digested food material will pass into the large intestine. Some indigestible plant products slow the rate of absorption of both sugars and fats.

Absorption in the large intestine

Very little save water is absorbed in the large intestine. It used to be imagined that poisonous substances such as histamine and tyramine, which certainly are made in the large intestine by the action of bacteria on *unabsorbed* amino acids, were absorbed into the blood stream and caused 'auto-intoxication'. This is a myth. All the theories and practices of patent medicine vendors, roughage enthusiasts, and nature cure folk, have no foundation in fact. The large intestine is not a cesspool poisoning the body and killing it before its time. In fact it has one function over and above that of acting as a dehydrator of and a reservoir for the unwanted or unabsorbed portions of food. That function is to act as an incubator of bacteria which manufacture various moieties of the vitamin B complex. These chemical substances pass into the fluid surrounding the bacteria and are absorbed into the blood stream. Consequently the production of these vitamins in the large intestine lowers the need for them by mouth; and anything which hurries material along the large intestine (purgatives, roughage, disease), and any drug which kills the bacteria, such as sulphonamides and the antibiotics, increases the need for these vitamins in the diet.

Metabolism

Proteins, then, are digested to amino acids and absorbed as such in the small intestine. Fats are partially digested to fatty acids and glycerol and absorbed in the same place. Some may be absorbed unchanged. Carbohydrates are digested to hexose sugars and, whereas it is likely that these are all absorbed in the small intestine, there is evidence that glucose can be absorbed also in the large intestine.

Carbohydrate metabolism

In discussing what happens to carbohydrates, i.e. when they are metabolised in the body, it is simplest to consider glucose, fructose and galactose. They pass into the blood stream, emerging from the intestines and perforce pass straight to the liver. All are stored there as glycogen, but some of the glucose passes on (perhaps all of it) and is transformed into glycogen in the muscles. Ultimately the glycogen is partitioned between the liver and the muscles. Storage of glycogen is encouraged by insulin, the internal secretion of the pancreas. Liver glycogen is readily transformed back into glucose whenever the blood sugar level falls below 0.08–0.06%, depending on the individual concerned. Fasting, cold and exercise, deprive the liver of glycogen, but not the muscles. It passes into the blood stream as glucose and is conveyed to the tissues—nervous system, glands and muscles—where it is consumed (oxidised) and energy obtained from this combustion. The final products of the combustion are carbon dioxide and water, but there may be more than one pathway (glycolysis and the 'pentose shunt' systems) used in the body. It is certain that the vitamins, thiamine, riboflavine and nicotinic acid are concerned in cellular combustion of carbohydrate to carbon dioxide and water, and also that insulin is essential somewhere in the process. Carbohydrates can be converted into fat and stored; the proportion so treated depends on the person—and on the quantity eaten.

Fat metabolism

Fats are absorbed partly as fat and partly as fatty acid and glycerol in the small intestine. The split fat is reconstituted in the intestinal epithelium and enters the blood, mainly via the lymph as droplets (*chylomicrons*) of neutral fat.

The fat is stored in the fat depots: under the skin, in the connective tissue of most organs, in the mesentery and around the kidneys. Heavy fat feeding also results in an increase of fat in the cells of the liver, even if carbohydrate is fed at the same time.

What happens to the fat when it is wanted to produce energy in the body is, today, being reconsidered. The neat little mathematical formula which has been held as truth, though with some misgivings, can no longer be accepted.

We used to believe that the body could not utilise fat except in the presence of glucose, and that if there were too little carbohydrate in the diet, or if it were unavailable, as in diabetes, the fat gave rise to acetone bodies, which were excreted partly as acetone in the breath but largely in the urine. These 'acetone bodies' are acetone, acetoacetic acid and β-hydroxybutyric acid. A person producing much of them is in the very uncomfortable state called ketosis, for acetoacetic acid is poisonous, causing headache, nausea and vomiting. Slight ketosis occurs in hunger and prolonged exercise, more marked ketosis in 'morning sickness', in cyclical vomiting and post-anaesthetic vomiting, and is very marked in advanced diabetes. Even mild diabetes when untreated may cause a ketosis.

It is perfectly true that if glucose be given to one with a ketosis, and in diabetes made available by insulin, that ketosis is cut to nothing. If a normal person has swung over into ketosis, cutting out fat from the diet and giving large amounts of carbohydrate will usually put an end to the trouble. To alleviate or cure morning sickness frequent meals mainly of carbohydrates are useful.

It is not astonishing that a theory was evolved that one had to have carbohydrates to help to metabolise fat and that fat, in the absence of carbohydrate is not utilisable in metabolism. In fact it seemed that one molecule of glucose could 'look after' two molecules of fat, and that, if there were not enough carbohydrate in the bloodstream, ketosis supervened and much of the energy derivable from fat was wasted.

This degree of precision is false. It is probable that some breakdown of glucose is needed to 'prime' the common oxidation pathways to both carbohydrate or fat, but this priming may also be performed by products of amino acid metabolism. Therefore the body *can* utilise breakdown products of fat in the absence of available carbohydrate. The diabetic *can* get about, though inefficiently. The obese person *can* take a diet with enormous amounts of fat in it which would cause ketosis in an average person. An obese person on a 4.2 MJ diet, 80% of the energy coming from fat and the rest from carbohydrate and protein, may show no ketosis. He must be metabolising fat, has little carbohydrate available and yet can oxidise fat.

Exercise on an empty stomach will produce a ketosis in the next one or two hours, but the ketosis will disappear if further exercise be taken. Clearly the muscles must be oxidising those ketone bodies.

It is almost certain that when fat is metabolised acetic acid (and not acetoacetic acid) is split off from the end of the fatty acid chain and the acetic acid thus produced is oxidised by the glucose oxidising system. Acetoacetic acid is a step in the *synthesis* of higher fatty acids, either from glucose or acetic acid and appears when this cannot be oxidised.

At present we have no pretty cut-and-dried theory to explain ketosis, and put in the place of that one considered correct and given in earlier editions of this book.

For the practical dietitian it is sufficient to note that the body works best if glucose (straight or from other carbohydrate) is available; that a diet with much fat in it may produce a ketosis in a normal person; that a ketosis is best treated by cutting down fat in the diet and increasing the carbohydrate and, in diabetes, making the carbohydrate available by insulin.

It is the brain and nervous system which demand glucose in the blood, they store no glycogen and do not use fat. The muscles are as efficient on fat as on carbohydrate, but utilise glycogen when they have to go in debt, temporarily, for oxygen.

Protein metabolism

The amino acids all pass into the bloodstream from the intestines and so inevitably go to the liver. They pass (at any rate in part) into the cells of the liver, which enlarge. None the less some pass on into the general circulation, for increase of amino acids in the blood has been definitely proved to follow a protein meal. It has been shown that if these amino acids are not accompanied by glucose a most detrimental, though perfectly physiological thing happens. There are enzymes in the liver which destroy the amino acids. The amino portion they remove and change into urea, which passes into the blood stream and is excreted in the urine—in other words valuable amino acids are lost to the body. After the amino group is removed the residue is changed either to glucose or to fatty acid, according to the nature of the amino acid. Leucine, phenylalanine and tryosine are changed to fatty acid and then to acetic acid; while alanine, glutamic acid and others change to glucose. The fatty acid and the glucose so formed are metabolised as sketched in the previous paragraphs. About 60% of the protein follows the glucose path and the rest the fatty acid path.

This raises a question. How then do the tissues ever get any amino acids to build up their substance? The answer is, they do not if protein is taken alone without any carbohydrate to accompany it. It has been shown that human beings may just as well starve themselves of protein if they do not accompany it with carbohydrate at the same meal. If breakfast consists solely of bacon or beef steak, and lunch of sugar and starch, and meals are like that alternately throughout the day, the body loses in the urine all the protein of the meals as nitrogenous substances plus all that lost when it is starving! So that if a person were to put himself rigorously on a Hay diet, which is supposed to divorce protein and carbohydrate in that diet, he might just as well starve himself of protein.

If carbohydrate be taken along with protein the amino acids arising from the protein get through the liver's gauntlet. It is supposed that the glucose inhibits the action of the deaminases, those enzymes which destroy amino acids. They escape their action, get into the general circulation and can be utilised for tissue-building purposes.

There is a continual interchange between the amino acids of the circulation and those of the tissues. Sometimes it is whole amino acids which are interchanged, sometimes it is the amino groups only, or sometimes the rest of the amino acid or perhaps only its COOH group, which changes place with that in the tissues.

In any case there will be amino acids in the blood, whether they come from the food directly or arise from the tissues as the result of interchange. These slowly disappear from the blood, tackled by the deaminases in the liver, changed to urea and excreted in the urine.

All the protein metabolism which is not more complicated than this is called *exogenous protein metabolism*, meaning by that term the metabolism of amino acids which have arisen directly from the protein eaten.

But, of course, that is not the end of the story. Some of the amino acids circulating in the blood are used to build up internal secretions, e.g. adrenaline, thyroxine and insulin, for example. These are oxidised or in some way got rid of after they have done their work. Some are used to manufacture creatine, essential in carbohydrate metabolism in muscle, and this substance in the form of creatinine is continually being lost to the body in the urine. Others are built right into the protein of the structures of the living cell. Still others are used to manufacture the nucleoproteins essential to the nuclei of cells. What happens to these afterwards we cannot as yet completely determine. The internal secretions form such a minute part of the problem that it is scarcely worth while to attempt to follow them up. The creatine we can adequately measure and its nitrogen form a large part of the total nitrogen excreted during starvation. We cannot follow the history of the amino acids built into the protein of the cytoplasm except by the means of isotopes, and what we learn suggests that when those amino acids leave the cytoplasm they are treated exactly as exogenous amino acids are treated. We can follow the amino acids built into nucleoprotein when, through wear and tear, they are discarded. The purine bodies which are the nitrogenous hall mark of the nucleoproteins, are synthesised from such amino acids as arginine and histidine, but when the time comes for their rejection they pass by a path altogether different from that of their synthesis. They are transformed by the liver to uric acid in man and excreted by the kidney, usually as sodium urate.

All this intimate metabolism of protein digestion products which have entered into chemical and cytological structures we term *endogenous nitrogen metabolism*—i.e. metabolism of the nitrogenous substances arising from within the cells. We can trace it only in part, through creatinine and uric acid estimations in the urine.

The chief importance of these considerations is seen in their relation to high protein feeding, and to the dietetic treatment of gout. In high protein feeding the end results are predominantly of exogenous origin. Now the changes which go on in the liver in the change of amino acids to fatty acid, glucose and urea, involve a wastage of heat which cannot be used for any purpose except maintenance of body temperature. Because we wear clothes and live in warmed houses this excess of heat is not used for maintenance of temperature, but is almost sheer waste. And it is therefore uneconomical to concentrate the consumption of protein into one meal in the day. Protein consumption should be spread well throughout the day's meals. The old-fashioned way of feeding public school pupils on a bread and butter breakfast and supper, plus a high protein midday meal, is to be condemned, and has been discarded.

5
Energy and nutrition

Until 1900 the energy content of foods dominated the science of nutrition. From then on, as the importance of the qualities of proteins, of vitamins and inorganic substances in foods loomed large, their energy content tended to be ignored. This was mistaken. Proper nutrition demands adequate supply of energy as well as of protein, vitamins and the inorganic materials. One without the other three is useless. From 1939 onwards, we have begun to feel differently and we now compare the energy-poor diet of poor people with the over-abundance of energy of the rich. We are right to worry about energy, for if the energy content of a diet is low, due to poverty, we can be sure that the proteins, inorganic substances and vitamins will be grossly deficient. Few foods are totally lacking in substances of these three constituents so if the energy content is abundant, then some protein etc. will be taken in as well. But *the energy producing foods must form the major part of the food we eat*. There is no way of avoiding the 500 g or so (1 lb in traditional weights) of solid food that must be eaten each day to provide our bodies with their essential energy. We may survive for long periods without enough protein, inorganic materials or vitamins, but we cannot last long without energy.

The units of energy

In nutrition the SI unit that is now preferred, and which will be used throughout this book is the *joule*. The joule was originally defined as the amount of energy expended when a force of 1 newton was exerted through a distance of 1 metre. It was an American armaments expert, employed by the Austrian Imperial Army who, nearly 200 years ago, originally showed that when physical force was expended, heat resulted, and Joule himself later determined the mathematical relationship between heat and physical force which is now enshrined in the modern use of his name for the basic energy unit. Heat energy used to be defined in separate units, *calories*. One calorie of heat raised the temperature of 1 ml of water through 1°C. We find that this is equal to about 4.186 joules. The joule is now used as the basic energy unit in mechanics, electricity and in heat. Therefore, in the study of energy turnover in the living body, and in that of the energy content of foods, the joule will be used here.

The reason for this link between physical force, chemical energy of food and heat, and for the ease with which scientists think of energy in all these forms in the same unit, the joule, is that energy, for all scientists studying the physical universe, from galaxies to our bodies and to simple chemicals, is the one fundamental thing. Energy can never (outside atomic nuclear reactions) be created or destroyed, only transformed. It may appear in many forms, as the kinetic energy of a rushing bullet or stream, the potential energy in water behind a dam, as electricity, light or heat, or in physical work. When a man walks upstairs, he does work (measured by his weight, multiplied by the height of the staircase). That work comes from energy liberated by oxidation of food in the body. If he is carried up in a lift, then the electrical energy, itself produced by oxidation of coal in the power station, does the work for him. Both the energy contained in his food and in the coal came from the sun. One could write the following series of energy transformations:

nuclear energy→heat and light→chemical energy in plants→food or coal
food→chemical energy in muscles→mechanical work
coal→heat→electricity→mechanical work

Since energy cannot be lost, only transformed, a definite amount of work must equal a definite amount of heat energy which, in turn, must equal a definite amount of chemical or electrical energy and so on. It is useful also to remind ourselves that the unit of electrical energy consumption, the *watt* is also clearly linked to the joule. Something using electrical energy at 1 joule/second is using 1 watt of electricity. The rate, then, of energy use of our typical man, 11 MJ/day, is about 100 joules/second or 100 watts. Just feel the heat given off by a 100 watt light bulb and then remember that you are giving off as much yourself.

During a normal day's activity a 'typical' adult man requires about 11 million joules of energy (11 MJ), all of which must come from his food and drink. If the energy content of the food is less than 11 MJ, then he raids the body energy stores (fat). If he eats more than 11 MJ some will be wasted, but some will be added to the energy stores in the fat depots. Each gram of fat contains 36 000 joules (36 kJ) of energy, so our typical adult, if he eats nothing can obtain all the energy he needs by using a mere 300 g (or 11 oz) of his stored fat. If he plays a vigorous game of squash he will raise his body temperature by 2°C, for almost all of the energy he uses appears within the body as heat (only 10–20% going into external work—hitting the ball and moving around the court). This temperature change would be caused by 588 kJ of heat, and the energy will be lost to the body, as he cools down to normal temperature after the exercise, in the air he breathes, in the evaporating sweat and to any cooler object in his environment. So the game of squash results in the extra loss of about 600 kJ, or 0.6 MJ, which is a small portion of his average daily energy used. This energy can be obtained from 17 g (less than 1 ounce) of fat.

As already mentioned, foods differ in their potential energy content. 100 g of bread contains 1.1 MJ of energy. That means that when it is eaten, digested and oxidised in the body, 100 g will produce 1.1 MJ, or about 1⅔ times the heat the squash player gained in his game. That game of squash cost the player about 60 g (or 2 oz) of bread. Energy contents of other typical foods are as follows: 100 g butter contains 3.1 MJ of energy, 100 g cheese 1.7 MJ, 100 g meat 1.3–1.8 MJ, 100 g potatoes 0.4 MJ, while 100 g cabbage or apples contain only 0.1 MJ of energy. So it *does* matter from the energy point of view what we eat. Bread, potatoes and vegetables are more bulky than butter, cheese and meat, so one has to eat more of them and one's appetite is more readily satisfied with a food intake of lower energy content than if one sticks to the energy-rich butter, cheese and meat.

The measurement of energy

The nutritional scientist has to know both the energy production rates of the living body when performing various activities, and also the energy content that can be released from foods when they are taken into the living body. Various methods have been devised, direct and indirect, to obtain these values.

The human calorimeter

The word *calorimeter* is applied to any apparatus that measures heat production, the word deriving from the Latin word *calor*, which means heat. Thus the word is still appropriate even though we have abandoned the calorie as a heat unit. In the human calorimeter, the heat output of a living man is measured directly. This sounds simple in principle, but in practice is a most costly, difficult and boring enterprise. Only a very few human calorimeters have ever been built, the most famous from our point of view being that designed, built and used by Atwater and Benedict in the USA between 1891 and 1903. Some of the essentials of its construction are shown in Fig. 5.1. The calorimeter proper is a copper room 3 × 2 × 2 metres, surrounded by a zinc shell. This is further surrounded by two wooden shells. Supports between the calorimeter and the shells are of some heat insulating material. These construction details ensure that no heat is lost from the copper calorimeter to the surrounding laboratory. Heat loss from the calorimeter can *only* be to the iced brine that flows through the radiator tube, and it is determined by measuring the temperature of the brine before and after it passes through the radiator, by recording the rate of brine flow and knowing its specific heat constant (the amount of heat needed to raise a given volume or mass through a given temperature range). A door and a window allow access to the calorimeter chamber, which contains bed, chair, table and apparatus for doing exercise. Fresh oxygen-containing air of the ideal temperature and humidity is supplied by the circuit shown in the diagram. Food and drink are handed in through the window. Urine and faeces must be handed out through the window.

Such apparatus is costly to build and to run. It takes several skilled technicians to run it and cannot be used whenever we wish to measure a person's energy output. This must be done by indirect means.

I have already mentioned the chemical energy contained in foods. This energy is liberated and, ultimately, transformed to heat, by the oxidation of foods or of body fat and glycogen stores, originally obtained from food.

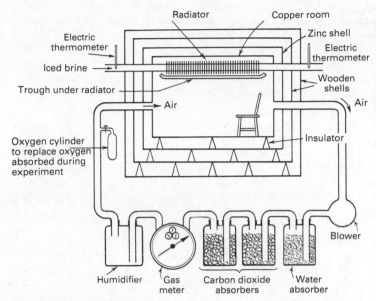

Fig. 5.1 The human calorimeter.

However it is performed, when a known amount of any chemical reacts with a known amount of oxygen, it will produce a known amount of heat, energy and carbon dioxide. In the laboratory these relationships can be determined by using the apparatus known as a *bomb calorimeter*.

The bomb calorimeter

This is shown in Fig. 5.2. It is a steel vessel which can be closed with a tight-fitting stopper. It contains a platinum crucible into which a weighed amount of combustible material (pure chemical or food) can be placed. It is filled with pure oxygen under pressure. The food can then be ignited by an electric current, when it will burn explosively. Before ignition the whole is sunk in a stirred water bath, of known volume and temperature, and the food is only fired when the temperature is constant. The heat of combustion is determined from the rise in water temperature, the rate of its subsequent cooling and the specific heat of the calorimeter itself.

Fat and carbohydrates are oxidised to CO_2 and water in a bomb calorimeter, just as in a living body. Fats give 38–39 kJ/g and carbohydrates 17 kJ/g, when oxidised in the bomb calorimeter, all the energy appearing at once as heat. In the body, oxidation proceeds in a series of separate chemical reactions; about half the energy is trapped in the 'high energy compounds' and may then be used for the many other reactions that require an input of energy before they can take place. These include muscular contraction.

In a bomb calorimeter, protein burns to water, CO_2 and oxides of nitrogen or nitric acid. This is highly poisonous, so, in the body, protein oxidation stops short of oxidising the $-NH_2$ groups. These are converted to

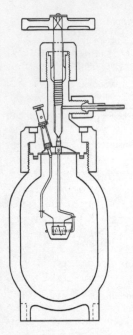

Fig. 5.2 The bomb calorimeter.

the harmless and soluble compound, *urea*. (Uric acid is similarly formed as the chief nitrogen-containing remainder of nucleic acids, present in all foods.) The bomb calorimeter can be used to determine the energy content of these substances, normally excreted from the body in urine. The difference, then, between the bomb calorimeter energy value for protein, and the energy value of the urea etc. derived from that protein gives the energy available from the oxidation of protein in the living body. This is 17kJ/g, the same as the value for starch or glycogen, by a happy coincidence.

The respiratory quotient (RQ)

By drawing up properly balanced chemical equations, as shown here, one can see that in oxidation of carbohydrates, the volume of CO_2 produced equals the volume of O_2 consumed. When fat is oxidised, however, the volume of CO_2 produced is about 70% of the volume of O_2 consumed. This is usually expressed as a decimal fraction, CO_2 produced/O_2 consumed and we say that the RQ for carbohydrates is 1.0 and that for the fat example shown below is 43/60 = 0.717. Other fats will have slightly differing RQs, depending upon the precise nature of their fatty acids.

Glucose oxidation

$$C_6H_{12}O_6 + 6O_2 \rightarrow 6H_2O + 6CO_2 + 15.5 \text{ kJ/g energy}$$

Starch oxidation

$$(C_6H_{10}O_5)_n + 6nO_2 \rightarrow 5nH_2O + 6nCO_2 + 17 \text{ kJ/g energy}$$

Fat oxidation (e.g. the chief fat of butter, glyceryl butyro-oleostearate)

$$C_3H_5O_3.C_4H_7O.C_{18}H_{33}O.C_{18}H_{35}O + 60 \ O_2 \rightarrow 43 \ CO_2 + 40 \ H_2O + 39$$
kJ/g energy

The non-nitrogenous portions of amino acids are, on the whole, intermediate in composition between fats and carbohydrates, and for protein the RQ is usually given as 0.81.

Finally, from these equations, one can emerge with figures for the energy produced for each litre of oxygen consumed in these oxidation reactions. Table 5.1 sets out the values for oxidising pure chemicals, carbohydrates, fats and proteins, and Table 5.2 extends further the energy production rates and the proportions of fat and carbohydrate oxidising at different RQs, once the energy production due to protein (the amount of which is determined from the rate of urea etc. excretion in the urine) has been determined.

Before concluding this section it must be emphasised that all these relationships are matters of pure chemistry and have all been determined in the laboratory. However, chemical relationships are the same in the living body as in the chemist's apparatus and we can apply the values for energy production from food oxidation that were obtained by chemists nearly a century ago, to studies of human energy needs and production today. This means simply that if one knows either the foods consumed or the respiratory gaseous exchanges, one can calculate the energy transformations in the body. The methods are generally known as *indirect calorimetry*.

Table 5.1 The energy obtained by oxidising foodstuffs (Zuntz, 1897).

	O_2 needed ml/g	CO_2 produced ml/g	RQ	Energy released kJ/g	Energy released per litre of O_2 used kJ
Starch	830	830	1.0	17.0	21.1
Glucose	747	747	1.0	15.5	20.8
Fat	2020	1430	0.71	39.0	19.6
Protein	966	782	0.81	18.6	19.3

Table 5.2 The energy produced and foodstuffs oxidised at different RQs.

Non-protein RQ	kJ per litre O_2	% Energy derived from Carbohydrate	Fat
0.71	19.6	1	99
0.75	19.8	16	84
0.80	20.1	33	67
0.85	20.3	51	49
0.90	20.6	68	32
0.95	20.8	84	16
1.00	21.1	100	nil

Respiratory gas measurements

The simplest indirect calorimetric method is that of measuring the rate of O_2 consumption using a *recording spirometer*. This is simply a gas holder containing oxygen, from which a person can breathe. The expired air is returned to the spirometer, after the CO_2 he has produced has been removed. The volume contained in the spirometer falls, and the rate of fall is recorded and measured, to give the rate of oxygen consumption. It is common practice then to assume that each litre of O_2 used causes the production of 20 kJ of heat and so the energy production can be simply calculated. Until the early 1970s such recording spirometers were becoming increasingly complex and expensive, but now a relatively cheap and simple apparatus has been produced, designed for secondary school use. It is depicted in Fig. 5.3. The main disadvantage of recording spirometers is that it is scarcely possible to study people in any other than stationary or resting situations. Furthermore one can obtain no information about the foodstuffs being oxidised, since measurements of CO_2 production and calculation of RQ are not made. The method depends also on the subject breathing regularly, equal volumes in each inhalation and these coming at regular intervals. A sigh or cough, even swallowing saliva, can disturb the record for as long as a minute. Most recording spirometers must be refilled after 10–15 minutes.

Early in the twentieth century, the collection, measuring and analysis of expired air was established by Haldane and Douglas at Oxford. Large rubberised canvas bags, holding 75–150 litres were used to collect the air. After a measured period of time the air in the bag could be mixed, a sample taken for analysis, and the volume determined. Bags could be carried on their backs by people employed in various activities, though the bulk of a filling 150 litre bag interferes considerably with activities such as cutting or loading coal at a mine's coal-face. In the 1940s and 1950s two devices were developed which have partly replaced the bag technique. The Kofranyi-Michaelis respirometer is a small mechanically-driven gas meter and sampling device, that measures the volume of the expired air and, also by a mechanical drive mechanism, takes a proportion of the air into a sample container for subsequent analysis. The IMP (Integrating Motor Pneumotachograph) machine does the same, but volume measured and sample collection are performed electrically. The whole apparatus is smaller and lighter than the K–M machine

All these methods depend finally on the chemical analysis of the expired air and the volume breathed in a known time. From the differences in O_2 and CO_2 composition of the expired air and of atmospheric air, the volume of the expired air and the time taken for its collection, the volumes of O_2 and CO_2 used or produced, and thence the metabolic rate, can be determined. If the urine formed during the same period is collected, its nitrogen content found, then the quantities of carbohydrate, fat and protein oxidised during this period can be determined.

Any method of expired air collection entails carrying a rubber or plastic mouthpiece and wearing a noseclip or plugs, or wearing a face-mask, and

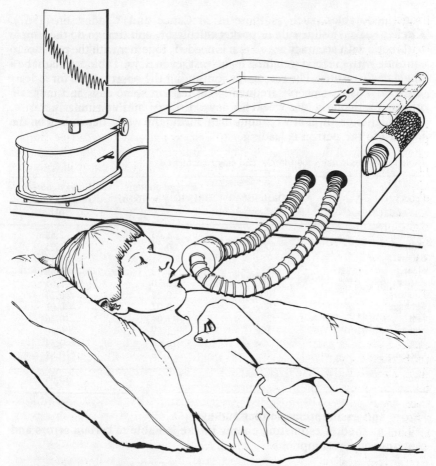

Fig. 5.3 The recording spirometer.

carrying douglas bags or other measuring/sampling devices. No one is able or willing to undergo this for long periods, and the analysis of many gas samples, by whatever means, can be a tedious job. These methods have been used, though, for measuring the energy costs of many different sorts of occupation, from lying asleep to work at the coal face or strenuous athletic pursuits. If a person can keep an accurate diary of his daily activities, it is possible, by referring to results of these studies, to determine approximately his daily energy expenditure.

Diet surveys

An alternative indirect way of measuring the energy output of a person is to determine his energy intake as food. The quantity of each food eaten during the period of study must be recorded, and its energy content determined from food tables, such as those of McCance and Widdowson (1967). Kitchen scales, a slide rule or pocket calculator, and time to do the simple arithmetic with accuracy are all that is needed, together with the patience to continue with the food weighing for at least seven days. Table 5.3 might be a single day's results. The reason for continuing the observations for at least seven days is that people frequently eat less on some days and more on others, particularly the weekend days. Energy output similarly varies, being higher or lower at weekends than during the week, depending on the sort of life the person is leading.

Table 5.3 A single day's food intake and energy content.

Food	Quantity	Energy content MJ/100g or 100ml	Energy content of day's intake MJ
Bread	250g	1.03	2.58
Milk	500ml	0.25	1.25
Bacon	75g	1.51	1.14
Meat	125g	1.32	1.65
Butter	50g	3.10	1.55
Potatoes	100g	0.24	0.24
Cabbage	100g	0.07	0.07
Jam	25g	1.04	0.26
Sugar	50g	1.59	0.40
Egg	50g	0.68	0.34
Cheese	50g	1.76	0.88
Total			10.36

Errors and assumptions in diet surveys

This method of estimating energy intake is liable to certain errors and contains some assumptions.

(1) That the tables consulted give the energy content of the various foods as cooked, or otherwise prepared, for eating, and not as purchased. For some it is the same, but for others the values can be very different.
(2) That food is not wasted by sticking to plates and other utensils after it has been weighed. In fact, there may be a 5% loss due to this factor.
(3) That the body absorbs from the gut all the food eaten. In fact, 5% of fat and 8% of protein is not absorbed, while absorption of digestible carbohydrate is virtually complete.
(4) That the person being studied is neither gaining nor losing body weight. This can be checked, but the water content may vary by 1–2 litres from day to day.
(5) That the energy values of foods, determined by the bomb calorimeter method, have made due allowance for their non-digestible (but combustible) carbohydrate or fibre content.
(6) That the conservations of matter and energy are true for the human body.

This last point was settled by direct human calorimetry studies. While the heat output from the people in the calorimeter was directly measured, the bomb calorimeter energy contents of all foods eaten and the excreta produced were determined. The energy intake then is the difference between these last two. Averaging many experiments, each lasting several days, it was found that the differences between energy output (heat) and energy input (food − excreta) were about ±0.2%. Thus, accepting the limits of the experimental errors of the methods, the conservation of energy is true for man, and we can accurately determine energy output, over periods of several days, by using the relatively convenient and simple method of estimating energy input from the food consumed. This method thus complements the respiratory gas methods, already described, which are most suitable for measuring metabolism in short periods of minutes or, occasionally, a few hours. By using the two indirect methods together we can determine the various metabolic needs of people at different ages and in differing states.

Group dietary surveys

Families or other groups of people can be studied, just as can individual people, and energy value of their food intake found. All foods that go onto the table are weighed before the meal, left-overs and wastage weighed after the meal, and the energy content of the difference found as already described. In such surveys on groups it is less easy to avoid *made-up* dishes. It will then be necessary either to obtain the recipe and estimate the energy content of each component separately, also allowing for water loss, when appropriate, in cooking, or to use the nearest equivalent dish that has been included in the food tables. Bomb calorimetry of the dish is beyond the resources of most workers.

A second method is the *housekeeping* one. A knowledge, at the beginning and end of a period, of all foods in store, and of all food bought during the period, can be used to determine the energy value of all the foods eaten during this period. Where accurate estimates of a country's agricultural imports, home production and export of food can be obtained, this method can be used to assess the energy available to a whole nation.

A third, much less accurate, method is the *budgetary* method. If one knows a family's total financial income, and expenditure on rent or mortgage, rates, fuel bills etc., one can determine how much is available for expenditure on food for the members of the family, and whether or not this provides sufficient food for their energy requirements. This must vary with the food prices in the available markets, but the minimum cost of an adequate diet can easily be determined (p. 143) and compared with the actual expenditure.

Basal metabolism

This is the metabolic activity needed to maintain a living body in the resting state, and when food is not being absorbed from the gut, that is 12–16 hours after the last meal. It is usually determined from a measurement of O_2 uptake using a recording spirometer, assuming an RQ of 0.85 and negligible protein metabolism, or an energy equivalent of 20 kJ/litreO$_2$. Basal metabolism is expressed as the joules produced per hour per square metre of skin surface (the basal metabolic rate or BMR). There is no good theoretical reason for relating metabolism to skin surface area, but in practice this gives a more constant value (for both human beings and many other mammals) than any other physical body measurement that can be simply determined. Skin area itself is related to a person's height and weight and can be determined from them by using lines I, II and III of the nomogram in Fig. 5.4. It is possible that skin area varies with metabolism because both vary with the *active cell mass* of a living body. This is the mass of actively metabolising tissue, so is equivalent to the whole body, less the deposits of fat, the crystalline material of bone and relatively noncellular connective tissues, tendons and ligaments. It is far harder to determine active cell mass than skin area. Figure 5.4 shows, in line IV what the BMR *ought to be*, in kJ/m^2/h, at different ages. The phrase *ought to be* really should read: *is found, on average, in healthy, well-fed but not overweight people to be*. A wide range of individual variation of 10–15% of this average value exists on both sides of the average. It is immediately apparent from this line that basal metabolism declines with age, and for any age is about 10% lower in females than in males. From lines III and IV one can then determine any person's total basal energy needs, taking account of his age, sex, height and weight. This nomogram does not apply for babies and children under 6 years of age. Soon after birth the BMR is 120, but rises rapidly, until at 6 years it is 240 kJ/m^2/h.

Knowledge of the BMR is important medically in detection of certain disease states. In human nutrition its importance is that it gives us a jumping-off point, below which a person's daily total metabolism can never fall, and below which therefore, the energy content of the food eaten cannot fall without eventual harm. For the average adult European male this is about 7.0 MJ/day. He needs, therefore, at least 7.0 MJ in his food each day if he is merely to exist and not actually *do* anything, even eat, digest and absorb this food! If any person's average food intake contains less than 7.0 MJ/day, then he *must be* undernourished.

During the normal living and working day we expend considerably more energy than this, and the more advanced textbooks of nutrition contain tables showing the estimated average energy needs of people in various occupations, and the energy needs of their leisure-time activities. One such estimate might be as follows:

Basal metabolism for 8 hours' rest in bed	2.34 MJ
Metabolism for leisure-time activities	3.12 MJ
Metabolism for 8 hours' moderate physical work	7.02 MJ
Total	12.48 MJ

This is this person's output. Allowing for a 5% loss from wastage at table

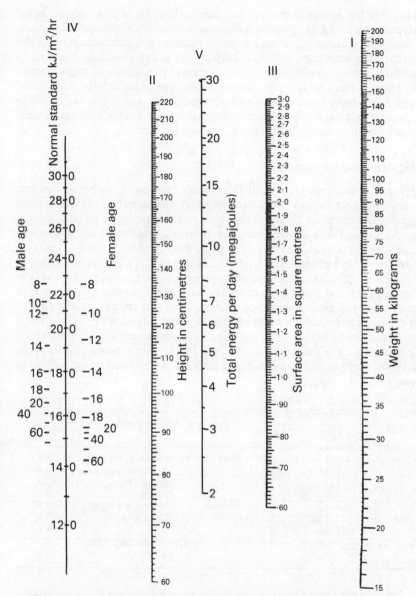

Fig. 5.4 The metabolic rate nomogram. The weight in kilograms is shown on Scale I. The height in centimetres is shown on Scale II. The surface area in square metres is shown on Scale III. The normal standard kilo joules per square metre of body surface per hour are shown on Scale IV. The total kilo joules per day are shown on Scale V.

Directions.—Keep the chart flat. Use a flexible ruler with a straight edge, made of perspex if obtainable or a strip of stiff paper such as a postcard. (A) Locate the position of the weight and height on Scales I and II respectively. Apply the straight edge of the ruler and note where it cuts Scale III. Read the figure on Scale III, which will give the surface area of the body in square metres. (B) Locate the surface area on Scale III, and the normal standard kilo joules per square metre per hour for the age and sex of the subject on Scale IV. Apply the straight edge of the ruler, and see where it cuts Scale V. Read this figure, which gives the total basal mega joules per 24 hours.

By permission from Price, 'Textbook of Medicine' (Oxford Medical Publications) and another 5% loss in digestion, this means that this person's input, in his food, must be 13.73 MJ per day on average. Similar calculations, based on the many measurements made by the respiratory gas estimations of all the different daily activities, and on accurate daily activity records, are used to determine the required intake for all sorts and conditions of men, women and children from which the various scales and standards of nutritional energy needs have been determined. By comparison of these, in individuals, groups or even whole nations, with the food available and consumed, one can instantly detect evidence of undernutrition.

Scales of energy needs

These are now prepared by official bodies, taking, it is hoped, expert advice, and, it is equally hoped, used in policy decisions by government and other organisations in their planning as is appropriate. The one quoted here, in Table 5.4 is drawn from the British Department of Health and Social Security (DHSS), having been published by them in 1969. This table differs from the American NAS table shown in earlier editions of this book, the American table tending to be more generous, particularly in first year of life and in the teens. Since such a table is drawn up by a panel of experts with considerable practical experience in many fields, it should be somewhere near the average requirement for each group, but should never be applied in hard and fast ways to individual people. Nor should such a table be regarded as immutable truth, to apply for all time. *It is the best estimate*, made in the late 1960s, *using the evidence then available*. It can be used in the following ways.

Table 5.4 The recommended daily energy intake for the UK (DHSS, 1969).

	Age	MJ			MJ
Children	0–1	3.3	Men	Sedentary	11.1
	1–3	5.5		Moderately active	12.4
	3–7	7.1		Very active	15.1
	7–9	8.8		Retired	9.3
Boys	9–12	10.5	Women	Most occupations	9.2
	12–15	11.7		Very active	10.5
	15–18	12.6		55–75	8.6
Girls	9–18	9.6		3–9 months pregnant	10.0
				Lactating	11.3

If a group of people—say an institution—is taking a diet within a ± 10% range of the appropriate estimated need, their diet may be considered satisfactory, *so far as energy is concerned*. This, of course, is where the housekeeping method of dietary survey is used, and one must be aware of the errors liable to occur in this method. Thus is one such survey in a school, the energy intake during the test period was found to be well *above* the estimated requirement. It was assumed that the school's catering manager, in order to impress his observers, had deliberately saved up foods from previous weeks in order to put on a good show during the test period!

In smaller groups—a family, for example—the individual diet survey method is used. An example is shown in Table 5.5, and the observed values are compared with the DHSS estimates.

Table 5.5 Actual energy intakes for a family

	DHSS estimate (MJ)	Actual consumption (MJ)
Father (bank manager)	11.1	13.0
Mother (moderately active)	9.2	10.8
Daughter 16 years old	9.6	5.0
Son 11 years old	10.5	9.0
Daughter 9 years old	8.8	9.2
Total	49.2	47.0
Total by Housekeeping Method		51.0

While it seems, at first glance at the total figures, that all is well, when one looks at the individual members of the family, some anxiety may be felt. Both parents are eating well above their estimated needs. Are they overweight, or more active than their job descriptions state. For instance, the bank manager may be a keen landscape gardener in his spare time. Then the actual intake of the 16-year old daughter gives cause for concern. Is this an expression of the anxiety over examinations that upsets many of her age? Is she having 'boyfriend trouble' or is she suffering from anorexia nervosa, a compulsive state in which the person (usually a 'high-achiever', late teen-aged girl) refuses to eat an adequate amount of food.

There is such a wide range of actual intake in normal healthy people, that it is only when the discrepancy between the observed intake and the estimated requirement exceeds 30% of the estimate (as it does in the 16-year-old girl just quoted) that further investigation is needed. Studies of large numbers of actual intakes, to obtain a reliable estimate of spontaneous variation are naturally very tedious to perform. Such a study was performed by McCance and Widdowson in the 1930s. 63 men and 63 women were studied by the individual method. They were of different ages and occupations, all were healthy and had an income such that no stinting of food was likely to occur. Nothing but their own appetites guided the food they ate. The average intake for the men was 12.6 MJ/day and for the women 9.25, in close agreement with the 'moderately active' figures in the DHSS estimates. But these averages were based on very wide ranges. The lowest intake for the men was 7.5 MJ and the highest 21 MJ. These figures indicate a frequency distribution curve that is skewed markedly towards the higher values, so the usual statistical measure of variation, the standard deviation, cannot be applied to the results. Incidentally, the man with the intake of 7.5 MJ was overweight and his weight was steady, and the one eating 21 MJ was of normal weight for his height and age. To vary from the average is in the nature (or cussedness?) of man!

Dr Widdowson (1951) has conducted a similar survey of 1000 children, over the age range 1–18 years. The results are shown in Table 5.6, compared with the DHSS estimates, and portrayed in Fig. 5.5. In the table the starred values are the ones that differ from the estimates by more than 10%. Throughout most of these results, excessive consumption, except in the first two years, occurs sporadically, and deficient intake was never seen. In the first two years, however, when parental pressure is most strongly applied, the observed intakes in both boys and girls, were considerably higher than estimated needs. Mothers have perhaps been obsessed with the need to produce chubby babies for the clinic and baby shows! What is quite unknown, but suspected, is that this pattern of overfeeding may set the scene for difficulty in restricting intake to match needs later in life, the consequence of which is obesity (of which more later).

Table 5.6 Actual energy intakes of children and estimated needs (MJ/day).

Age	Actual intakes		Estimated needs	
	Boys	Girls	Boys	Girls
1	4.8*	4.8*	3.3	
2	5.8*	5.8*	5.0	
3	7.1*	6.3	5.9	
4	7.6*	7.1	6.7	
5	7.2	7.1	6.7	
6	8.0	8.3*	7.5	
7	9.2*	8.3*	7.5	
8	9.2	8.7	8.8	
9	10.2*	9.1	8.8	
10	10.4	9.7	10.5	9.6
11	10.5	9.6	10.5	9.6
12	10.9	9.8	10.5	9.6
13	11.5	10.4	11.7	9.6
14	12.5	10.9*	11.7	9.6
15	14.2*	10.8*	11.7	9.6
16	12.9	9.8	12.6	9.6
17	13.3	10.4	12.6	9.6
18	14.2*	10.4	12.6	9.6

Once again the individual figures, from which the averages were calculated, showed great variability. Thus in any one age group a child might be found taking twice the amount of energy taken by another in the group. One cannot say, if both were healthy otherwise, that one was eating too much or the other too little. Once again, these figures show that in using estimated scales or recorded intakes in studies of (or in the forward planning of) meals for individuals, the scales or results cannot be rigidly applied. They can be applied to large groups only. This is not to say that they can never be used on the individual basis. Each considerable departure from the average should be examined in relation to health and activity. It may mean nothing—it usually does—but it may be a pointer to some maladjustment in body or mind. Similarly the dip at 16 seen in both sexes in Dr Widdowson's results

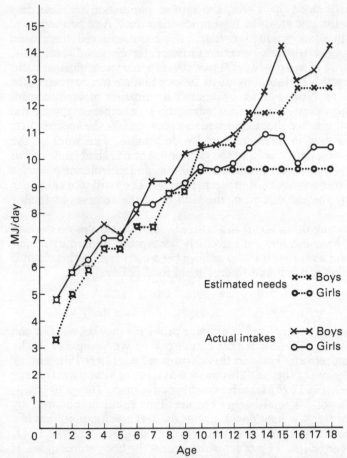

Fig 5.5 Actual energy intakes of boys and girls of different ages compared with DHSS estimates of energy needs.

may be related to examination or school-leaving problems. Finally, one must speculate about how truly representative of British youth were her 1000 children.

The global position

However many doubts and reservations we may have when applying these scales to individuals or small groups in Great Britain or other similar states, when they are related to the world at large, no one will deny that the situation is critical. If we accept the figures collected by the FAO as substantially correct, we see that at least half of the world's population suffers from a marked energy deficit, and that less than a quarter obtain a food intake that is really adequate. Moreover, due to improved medical care, particularly since the 1940s, the rate of population increase may actually exceed the rate at which food production rises. And furthermore, the increases in food production that have been achieved have been obtained by using exhaustible reserves of mineral fertiliser and fossil fuels, and at the expense of soil quality and tree cover in many marginal and arid regions of the earth's surface. Optimists believe that we can overcome, for all time, these problems, aided by a strict application of birth-control measures. The present writer must admit he is numbered among the pessimists and thinks we should prepare and plan *now* for the spectre, first foreseen by Malthus in 1798, of world-wide famine. The work of the optimists on raising crop yields, in the greater use of marginal land, and in the provision of tube wells, mineral fertiliser, and petroleum fuels for agricultural machinery, are all short-term policies. They will sooner or later be overtaken by the exhaustion of the land or of the reserves of fuel or fertiliser.

Whatever we may think about the future though, the scales do provide clear evidence, here and now, of extremely widespread undernutrition in the world and the use of such scales as have been discussed in this chapter forms the basis of national and international food policy.

Obesity

Whatever the actual or predicted worldwide problems may be, a major one that faces us in the UK now is that of the person whose energy intake exceeds his requirement. Early in this chapter we considered the energy cost of a typical game of squash. This was 0.6 MJ, out of a daily total energy turnover of, perhaps, 12 MJ for a reasonably active man. The game, then, accounts for 5% of his total energy output. This could be obtained by oxidising 17 g of fat. We must now consider the reverse situation, that of a person whose intake is 12 MJ, but whose energy output is only 11.4 MJ. The rest is converted into 17 g of fat which enters the body stores of fat. If this happens every day of a year, the person will be 365 × 17 g, = 6.2 kg heavier at the end of the year than he was at the beginning. In 10 years, if he were to continue with only this 5% imbalance between input and output, his weight might be doubled!

While this extreme situation may happen only rarely, minor degrees of obesity are so common that we hardly notice them. But every increase in weight, 'the middle-aged spread', a 'beer-pot', call it what you will, carries with it penalties. The heart, circulatory and respiratory systems all have to work that much harder to maintain and move the extra weight around. Their reserves to deal with exercise or acute illness are correspondingly reduced. The bearing surfaces at the joints between the bones—particularly in the lower spine and in the legs—are overloaded and may wear down, causing arthritic changes which further embarrass activity. The overweight have an increased incidence of such diseases as diabetes and arterial disease. We do not know why, but every life insurance company recognises that to be obese reduces one's chances of leading a long and healthy life.

The control links between energy needs of a living body and its energy intake in food are still unknown, despite much energetic research into this very important subject. Many people have hoped to show that needs control intake, but none of the experiments designed to demonstrate this at the sort of level described above, for the balance must be better than 5% or even 1% in the long term, have identified the control mechanism. I have often wondered whether, while a 'coarse' adjustment may work in this way through a feeding centre in the brain, which is identified and which appears to be sensitive to blood glucose concentration, the 'fine' adjustment operates in the reverse direction, the body's oxidative rate rising and falling as food intake increases or decreases. Even if this were so, we would have to establish a cause–effect link between the food intake and the overall level of oxidative activity of all cells before any physiologist, nutrition scientist or doctor would accept such a speculation. In any case, the evidence from all the overweight men, women and children in the UK nowadays shows that any such 'fine control' mechanism is not particularly effective when intake exceeds needs by a small amount, but steadily over a long period of time. You should remember that a 1% imbalance every day may lead to the deposition of over 1 kg of fat in a year, and that the most effective way of removing this extra fat is by ensuring that intake remains lower than requirement, consistently over many weeks or months. Maintaining a constant body weight is not so much a medical emergency, more a way of life!

6

Foods eaten chiefly for their energy content

In truth, of course, and excluding only white sugar, cooking fats and oils and alcoholic distillates, no food eaten has a single function in nutrition. Most foods provide energy, proteins, vitamins and essential inorganic materials, so the separation into three parts of what used to be a single, 53-page chapter on the nature of foods (which came as a somewhat indigestible dessert at the end of earlier editions of this book) is somewhat arbitrary and foods will have to be mentioned in more than one place. However, the first mention will usually be the most detailed and cross references will be provided as appropriate.

The classification of foods used here is by function in nutrition, not by their biological kingdom or sub-classification. In this chapter, now that we have established the energy needs of people, we will determine how best these needs can be satisfied. The chemicals that are eaten primarily to provide energy are the fats and the carbohydrates, and it is foods containing these that will now be described.

Foods containing oils and fats

Chemically, the biological oils and fats are very similar, for an oil is simply a fat that is liquid at room temperatures. Their energy values are almost identical. (The biological oils must be distinguished from medicinal liquid paraffin oil better known in the USA as mineral oil, which is not a glyceryl ester of fatty acids, but a mixture of paraffin hydrocarbons that form a slow-flowing liquid at room temperature. Chemically it is like petrol.) Fats and oils are the most concentrated food source of energy. Their consumption has risen greatly since the nineteenth century and, even during the great depression of the 1930s, exceeded 100 g/person/day. This provides nearly 4 MJ energy or about 40% of the average daily need. It can be a cheap source of energy, too. Thus in the 1930s, when margarine was priced at 5 d/lb (in SI and new currency units, 0.5 p/100 g), it provided more energy per penny than any other food.

Butter

Butter has, by tradition for over 100 years, been regarded as the most esteemed fat. At its current price of 10 p/100 g (25 p/½ lb), it provides 0.3 MJ/1 p. Butter is made from the fat of milk. This is first partially soured, to de-stabilise the emulsified fat particles and then churned so that these particles adhere to each other. It is the specific bacteria that sour the milk that impart the flavour to butter, though this can be mimicked by acetylmethylcarbinol and diacetyl. The finished product is a water-in-oil emulsion, containing about 14% water and 0.4% of milk protein. The colour is due to carotene pigments, and salt may be added to enhance its keeping quality.

Margarine

Margarine was devised in 1869 as a butter substitute. It was first prepared from waste beef and mutton fat (no longer needed for candle making), but is now prepared from various vegetable oils. The double bonds in some of the vegetable oil fatty acids have first to be hydrogenated, to provide a fat that will have the quality of butter at room temperature. The fat is then emulsified with soured skim milk and prepared for the market. Since the sources of fat, the various vegetable oils, are considerably cheaper than that of milk, margarines are also cheaper than butter, except where dairy farmers persuade governments to adopt a protectionist policy, as in the USA at one time and in the EEC in the 1970s. To the fat mixture of margarine, vitamins can be added, as will be described in Chapter 10. The compositions of butter and margarine are compared in Table 6.1.

Table 6.1 Compositions of butter and margarine (values per 100g).

		Butter	Margarine
Protein	(g)	0.4	trace
Fat	(g)	85.1	85.3
Carbohydrate	(g)	trace	nil
Calcium	(mg)	15	4
Iron	(mg)	2	3
Retinol	(μg)	720–1200	900
Cholecalciferol	(μg)	0.25–2.5	2–9
Energy	(MJ)	3.32	3.32

Cooking fats and oils

Cooking fats and oils are prepared from both animal and vegetable sources and are used, as the name suggests, almost exclusively in culinary processes. Lard, suet and vegetable cooking fat are bought in the butchers' and grocers' shops, while dripping is prepared in the home. Various vegetable cooking oils are also now available. Lard is prepared from pigs' fat depot tissue. It has a low melting point and is virtually 100% fat. Suet is the chopped or flaked fat depot tissue of the ox. A varying amount of rice flour is added to flaked suet to prevent the flakes sticking to one another. Its fat content may vary from 99% down to 70%. Dripping is the rendered fat that escapes from joints of meat while they are being cooked. If clarified it is virtually pure fat, and carries with it some of the flavour characteristic of its meat source. Vegetable-origin cooking fat, and the cooking oils are also pure fat. The energy content of the pure fats is 3.9 MJ/100 g. Where, as in butter, there is 14% water present, or, as in suet, rice flour, the energy values are lower, at 3.3 MJ/100 g and 2.7 MJ/100 g respectively.

Other fat-containing foods

Milk contains 3–6% fat, the amount varying with the breed of cow or other mammal from which the milk comes. Milk is unusual in that 11% of milk fat consists of acids with 4–12 carbons in the fatty acids, of which butyric acid (4 carbons) is the typical example.

Milk can be fractionated, concentrated and dried in various ways, with or without its fat content. These will mostly be described in the chapter on protein foods, though some that contain the fat will be described here.

Cream is a concentrate of the fatty portion of milk. Single cream has a minimum legal content of 18% milk fats and double cream a minimum of 48% fat. The 'top' of the milk as normally sold contains up to 20% fat.

Ice-cream as commercially prepared may contain 8–12% fat, which may originate from milk, or from a vegetable source.

Cheese is prepared from milk by precipitating the protein, casein, from its soluble precursor. The casein takes with it much of the fat originally present in milk, so cheeses may contain 20–40% fat, depending on their source.

Eggs contain about 12% of fat, concentrated in the yolk, which is about 30% of the whole egg. Therefore egg yolk is about 40% fat.

Some *fish* contain a considerable amount of fat. Chief among these are herrings, sprats and mackerel, which contain 8–15% fat, depending upon the species and the season. This fat can form an appreciable portion, then, of the energy content of the fish, though they will be more fully described in Chapter 8 on protein foods. The fat content of *mammalian and avian meat* also varies considerably, but in some species it may contribute substantially to the energy value. For example bacon contains up to 45% fat, while beef and lamb are about 30% fat, and veal only 17%.

Polyunsaturated fatty acids and cholesterol

In the 1960s many people began to accept the growing body of evidence that the unsaturated fatty acids were protective and that a high dietary intake of cholesterol was harmful. I am still not entirely convinced by the evidence for either statement. The level of cholesterol in the blood, which *may* have something to do with arterial disease, is only partly determined by the cholesterol in food, because, no matter what our dietary intake, we make cholesterol in our own bodies. Foods high in cholesterol are eggs and brains. A high intake of saturated fatty acids and fatty acids containing a single double bond raises plasma cholesterol, while increasing the intake of polyunsaturated fatty acids (those having two or more pairs of carbon atoms linked by double bonds) lowers plasma cholesterol. Most land animal fats, milk and its products ('every cow should carry a government health warning', so some say!) and some vegetable oils contain mainly saturated fatty acids, whereas fish and other vegetable oils contain larger amounts of unsaturated fatty acids, as is shown in Table 6.2.

Table 6.2 The fatty acid composition of some food fats.

Food	C4–12 Saturated	C14–18 Saturated	C16 + 18 1 double bond	C18 2 double bonds	Others 2 or more double bonds	1 double bond
Milk etc.	11	47	36	4	1	
Beef		53	44	2		
Pork		34	44	21		
Fish oil		23	27	7	43	
Coconut oil	58	31	8	2		
Corn (maize) oil		15	31	53	1	
Ground nut oil		15	55	30		
Olive oil		16	71	10		
Palm oil		45	45	9		
Rape seed oil		4	16	14	9	50
Soya bean oil		14	24	53	7	
Sunflower seed oil		11	25	63		

Apart from the fat fish, herrings, mackerel, salmon, we do not directly eat much of these materials. They can be used as cooking fats, though on exposure to heat and air the double bonds are said by some to be readily oxidised. They can be incorporated into margarine and such margarine is now marketed, though it is more costly than the cheapest butter. Attempts are also being made to persuade those animals we rear for their meat to incorporate more polyunsaturated fatty acids in their depot fat. This can be done by feeding them vegetable material or fish meal containing the unsaturated fats but in the interest of the global nutrition state, it would perhaps be better for these to be fed directly to humans. To summarise, *if* it is accepted that a high blood cholesterol is harmful, then this can be increased by saturated fatty acids and reduced by polyunsaturated fatty acids. The former are present in milk, meat, palm and olive oils, the latter in fat fish and the other vegetable oils in regular use, or coming into use in the 1970s. Their correct use in cooking and as a butter substitute is required if their intake is to be increased. Herring and mackerel, furthermore, must be protected from over-fishing if their continued supply is to be maintained.

Sugars and syrups

Sugar has, since the sixteenth century, become an important food commodity. The development, first of sugar cane and later of sugar beet cultivation, has been the cause. The average annual consumption in the UK today is 50 kg per person; 140 g/day. This provides 2.3 MJ, about 20% of the day's requirement. Such consumption alarms dietitians for they fear that, if the appetite is sated with sugar, then other foods will be crowded out of the diet. Furthermore it is possible that sugar may partly account for dental caries, diabetes and obesity.

Sucrose is the common form of sugar, used both in cooking and on the table. It is the same chemical substance, whether prepared from the sap of the sugar cane, or from the sugar beet root. The only reasons for choosing one rather than the other source (and cane sugar, even in a community with a labour force living at a high economic level, such as Queensland, costs less to produce than does beet sugar) are political and economic, not a matter of taste at all. Other sugars include malt sugar (maltose), milk sugar (lactose), grape sugar (glucose) and fruit sugar (fructose). All sugars provide about 1.6 MJ energy/100 g, and are among the cheapest sources of energy.

In the manufacture of crystalline sugar from cane sap or beet juice, *treacle, molasses and golden syrup* are produced. Due to the partial breakdown of sucrose to glucose and fructose, these compounds prevent the complete crystallisation of the sucrose. These syrups thus contain a mixture of sugars, together with a concentrate of other compounds present in the original sap. Their composition is given in Table 6.3.

Table 6.3 Composition of syrups (per 100g).

		Black treacle	Golden syrup
Protein	(g)	1.06	0.35
Fat		nil	nil
Carbohydrate	(g)	67.4	78.0
Calcium	(mg)	495	26
Iron	(mg)	9.2	1.4
Energy	(MJ)	1.07	1.24

Honey is a syrup made by bees from the sugary secretions of many flowers. It contains mainly a mixture of glucose and fructose, whereas plant nectars are mainly sucrose. The bee must therefore have digested the sucrose to the simpler sugars, or inverted it. The flavour and composition of honey are determined by the flowers that the bees collect nectar from, the locality and its weather. Examples are shown in Table 6.4. Honeys have no nutritional virtues, apart from their pleasant flavour, other than the energy content of about 1.2 MJ/100 g.

Table 6.4 Compositions of various honeys (per 100g).

		Honey 1	Honey 2	Honey 3	Honey 4
Protein	(g)	?	0.4	0.4	0.4
Fat	(g)	?	?	trace	nil
Sucrose	(g)	1.90	2.69 ⎫	76.40	68.80
Invert sugar	(g)	74.98	71.40 ⎭		
Dextrin	(g)	1.51	?	nil	?
Energy	(MJ)	1.21	1.16	1.19	1.15

Invert sugar is the equimolecular solution of glucose and fructose, formed by bees' invertase, or by boiling a sucrose solution in the presence of acid.

This occurs in both home and commercial jam-making, and the change contributes to the setting property of jam. It adds no nutritional value to jams, which, apart from the ascorbic content of some, are of value only for their energy content of about 1.04 MJ/100 g.

Liquid glucose is a substance widely used in the food manufacturing industry. It is formed by boiling starch solution with acid. It is used in making confectionery, beer and some jams. It contains 18% water, some dextrins and 68.8% of glucose. Its energy content is 1.32 MJ/100 g. Pure powdered glucose and drinks containing a high concentration of glucose are used to supplement the energy intake in ill-health. They should only be given upon doctors' orders. Boiled sweets and toffees are made from glucose and have energy values of 1.56 and 1.74 MJ/100 g respectively.

Maple sugar is used as a sweet-meat, but it is sucrose prepared from the sap of the North American tree, the sugar maple. In the boiling process a small amount of sucrose is changed to invert sugar.

Fresh fruit

Apart from the sucrose content of sugar cane, sugar beet and maple syrup, all fruits contain varying amounts of sucrose, fructose or glucose. Some of these are native to Great Britain, some have been brought over and cultivated here, and some have to be imported, frequently ripening on voyage.

Most fruits contain 3–15% carbohydrate and when ripe this is usually present as a mixture of fructose and glucose, often in equal amounts. Apples and pears contain mainly fructose, apricots and peaches mainly sucrose, while grapes contain up to 16% glucose. The energy content of fresh fruit therefore ranges from 0.06–0.3 MJ/100 g.

Many fruits are preserved, in sealed tins, bathed in a sugary syrup. Typical carbohydrate and energy values for the whole contents of such a tin would be 20 g and 0.32 MJ/100 g.

Dried fruits should be considered here since they provide energy only, due to their sugar content. These include currants, raisins and sultanas (made from different kinds of grapes), prunes, dried apricots and figs. Many have lost so much water that their energy content is around 1.0 MJ/100 g.

Alcohol

Alcohol is produced from maltose, glucose and fructose by micro-organisms, particularly by yeasts. In this process, the glucose molecule is internally rearranged and split into two fragments which become ethyl alcohol. No oxygen is required, and about 10% of the chemical energy of the glucose molecule is obtained by the yeast. The remaining 90% is retained in the alcohol molecules.

Maltose, containing two glucose molecules, is produced from the starch of grain seeds when they sprout. The other two sugars are present in fruit juices and in honey. Since prehistoric times all three sources have been used to produce alcohol-containing drinks. It is generally assumed that their development was due to the psychotropic action of the ethyl alcohol produced, and to their flavour, but since yeasts exist which produce an alcohol concentration too high to be tolerated by other micro-organisms, it could be argued that alcoholic fermentation is a means of preserving the larger part of the energy value of the original food material, at the cost of losing 10% to the yeast, and being intoxicated by the product!

While for most people nowadays alcoholic drinks form a negligible or small portion of our energy intake, this can be considerable in a person who becomes addicted to alcohol. In such a person, the alcohol alone may account for 50% of his energy intake, and if he takes it as sweet sherry, then he will also be ingesting a considerable amount of sugar as well.

One must remember that, while the grain derived brews contain some of the B group of vitamins, most alcoholic drinks (and all of the distillates prepared from them) contain energy alone, with no other substance of any nutritive value. The damage to liver and brain that results from excessive drinking throughout life is as likely to be due to absence of essential nutrients as it is to any toxic component of the alcoholic drink, while that to the stomach is an example of the direct toxic action of the alcohol or other substances formed during fermentation in small amounts. Since, in many people, alcohol is taken *in addition* to a normal diet, containing all the energy they need, their total energy intake is greater than their needs and they become fat.

One final point in favour of alcoholic drinks is that the pleasant taste of many is an appetite stimulant and a 'drink before a meal' may readily raise the amount of food eaten and properly digested by a sick or convalescent person, provided he has not got a stomach complaint.

Table 6.5 gives the composition and energy value of some alcoholic beverages.

Table 6.5 The composition of some alcoholic beverages (per 100 ml).

	Alcohol g	Protein g	Carbohydrate g	Calcium mg	Thiamine mg	Nicotinic acid mg	Energy MJ
Draught bitter	3.1	0.3	2.3	10.8	trace	0.70	0.13
Stout	4.3	0.3	2.1	4.8	trace	0.70	0.16
Sweet cider	3.7	trace	4.3	7.9	trace	0.07	0.18
Red wine	9.4	0.2	0.3	7.4	trace	0.15	0.29
White wine	8.8	0.1	3.4	14.1	trace	0.08	0.31
Dry sherry	15.7	0.2	1.4	7.1	trace	0.08	0.48
Sweet sherry	15.6	0.3	6.9	6.8	trace	0.15	0.57

Starch

This is the main carbohydrate store material in plants, though some produce an appreciable amount of fat in their seeds, as already mentioned, and one family of plants, the Compositae, which includes daisies, dahlias and artichokes, use a fructose polymer, *inulin*, in place of starch. Our digestive enzymes cannot hydrolise inulin, so most of its energy content is unavailable to us.

The principal sites of starch storage that we use for foods are seeds, principally of the grass family (known collectively as *cereals*), and of the legume family, the *pulses* or beans, roots and tubers (modified plant stems).

The cereals

These are collectively by far the most important food crop in the world's agricultural system. This is as clearly true today as it was in 1925 when the science fiction novel *Nordenholt's Million* by J. J. Connington was first published describing the effects of a world-wide failure of grain crops, as it was in Imperial Rome, dependent upon Egypt's wheat, and as it probably was at the very origin of human civilisation. The term should be applied to the seeds of members of the grass family (wheat, maize, barley, oats, rye and rice), but it is usually extended to include buckwheat and millet, even arrowroot, sago and tapioca which are not grass-seed products at all. The term is also used in reference to the various breakfast food products that we now eat instead of oat porridge.

Nutritionally, these foods are eaten for their starch content, supplying us with a large part of our energy needs. However, most of these foods contain up to 13% protein, vitamins, inorganic materials and some contain up to 8% fat. Cereals are essentially the energy source of the poor. Thus in Great Britain in the 1920s, wheat in one form or another supplied 60% of the energy intake of the working classes, the majority then of the population. The nearest corresponding figures for the 1970s are that in the whole UK wheat products supply only 26% of our energy intake. In poorer countries of the world 70–80% of energy intake is derived from a cereal substance.

However, cereals alone cannot supply all our nutritional requirements. Although 250 g (8 oz) of bread (a not unreasonable daily intake) supplies 20 g of protein, this protein is low in content of some of the essential amino acids (see Chapter 7). Cereals completely lack ascorbic acid and only yellow maize supplies any retinol. Most cereals are deficient in fats (oats and maize being the exceptions) and contain phytic acid which reduces the absorption of calcium and iron from the food.

The nutritional quality of cereals is further affected by the methods commonly used in preparing them for human consumption. These involve some process, usually milling, grinding or pounding, that breaks up the whole seed and enables the removal of the outer indigestible layers. In these processes, the parts containing much of the stored vitamin content may also be lost, though much of the phytic acid is also removed. The problems of the effects of these processes on the nutritional value of individual cereals will be discussed along with each of the separate types.

Wheat

This is usually regarded by western peoples as the king of cereals. It was first cultivated in the Middle East, so should be regarded as a sub-tropical plant. By breeding new varieties man has extended the cultivation of wheat into many different climatic conditions and, broadly speaking, two main species have emerged, *Triticum durum* and *Triticum vulgare*.

Figures 6.1 and 6.2 show the chief component parts of the wheat grain. There are four main parts:

(1) The germ, or embryo plant, forming 1.5–2% of the whole grain.
(2) The endosperm or kernel, two masses of nutrients for the use of the embryo plant, when it germinates or starts to grow. It forms about 85% of the whole grain. Its outermost layer is the protein-rich aleurone layer.
(3) The scutellum is a thin membrane separating germ from endosperm. Though less than 1% by weight of the whole grain it contains 60% of the thiamine (vitamin B_1) in the grain.
(4) The bran, which is the tough outer coat of the seed, containing cellulose and other indigestible materials. It forms 12–13% of the whole grain.

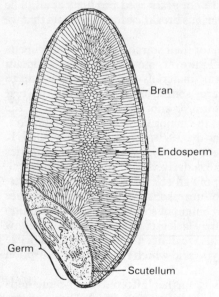

Fig 6.1 Section through a grain of wheat

The chemical composition of the chief components and of two types of whole grain wheats are shown in Table 6.6.

Bran is theoretically of nutritional value. It has more fat, calcium and iron than the whole grain. However 50% of its high phosphorous content is represented by phytic acid which blocks calcium and iron absorption. The high 'cellulose' content, which includes other non-digestible materials, may upset some peoples' digestive system, though since about 1970 evidence has been accumulating that shows that these materials may be of protective value against various diseases. They reduce the rate of glucose and fat

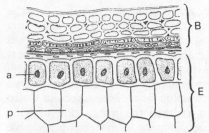

Fig. 6.2 Cross-section through the branny envelope and the outer portion of the endosperm.
B. Bran. E. Endosperm consisting of *a*, layer of aleurone cells; *p*, parenchymatous cells.

Table 6.6 Composition of wheat grains (per 100g).

		Bran	Endosperm	Germ	Whole English	Whole Manitoba
Water	(g)	8	13	8	13	13
Protein	(g)	10.9	13.1	32.0	9.1	13.9
Fat	(g)	4.2	1.2	7.7	2.3	2.6
Digestible carboyhdrate	(g)	54.5	71.6	37.8	68.1	64.3
Calcium	(mg)	98.0	13.0	58.0	36.0	28.0
Iron	(mg)	12.9	1.8	9.7	3.1	3.9
Thiamine	(mg)	nil	0.07	2.10	0.29	0.36
'Cellulose'	(g)	18.0	0.7	1.8	5.7	1.7
Phosphorus	(mg)	815	84	?	340	350

absorption after a meal and thus cut off the peaks in glucose and fat blood levels that may contribute to diabetes and artery disease. The consistency of the contents of the large bowel is softened and the material passes through more rapidly. These facts are thought by some to reduce diverticular disease, colonic cancer, haemorrhoids and varicose veins.

Endosperm is composed chiefly of starch and protein. It contains little fat, thiamine, calcium or iron. Its outer aleurone layer is rich in protein and vitamins of the B group.

The germ contains the highest percentage of fat and of protein. It also contains more vitamins, calcium and iron than does endosperm.

Table 6.5 shows also that Canadian wheat has somewhat more protein and thiamine than has the English wheat. *Triticum durum* varieties are also rich in protein. The higher protein contents make for a better risen loaf of bread and also enable the manufacture of different pasta varieties from *Triticum durum* flour. The protein in the aleurone layer, however, reduces the ability of bread dough to rise.

It can now be seen how the miller's, baker's and consumers' interest conflict with those of nutrition. People have come to prefer the smooth, white and light bread that can be made with pure endosperm flour of Canadian wheat which is, in any case, more easily handled by modern baking methods. Steel roller grinders and sieves can separate out the components of the wheat grain into bran, endosperm and germ, removing also the aleurone layer from the endosperm. Commercial white flour is virtually pure endosperm, representing about 70% of the original wheat grains, and therefore known as *70% extraction* flour. Normal wholemeal flour is 90% extraction flour, the coarser bran only being omitted, and true wholewheat flour is of course 100% extraction flour. In the second world war, the government of Great Britain ordered the production of 85% extraction flour, in order to save on shipping space. A perfectly acceptable bread, from the consumer's point of view, can be made from any of these flours. Wholewheat, wholemeal and 85% extraction flour will not keep as well as 70% extraction flour, because the fat may become rancid. I find that the high extraction breads, also perhaps because of their fat content, seem to be moister than 70% flour bread. I prefer their roughness and closeness of texture to the light, tasteless cotton wool of modern (1970s) white flour bread, and clearly remember first meeting the richly flavoured, moist 85% extraction bread on board a ship when returning to Britain from Canada in 1943. However, I am in a small minority, for 90% of the bread sold in the UK in the 1970s is made from white flour.

To get away from personal preferences (albeit important in *human* nutrition), to commercial and nutritional considerations, one has first to say that the 30% removed is not wasted. It can be fed to livestock and help produce meat, milk or eggs. It can be fractionated further and patent foodstuffs or vitamins of the B group prepared from it. The 70% extraction flour will keep better than the original grains, for it contains little fat, and lacks many food factors essential for the growth of pests, moulds etc. It is, as already seen, preferred by the baking business, and, it would seem, by the naive consumer. It is lacking, as has already been mentioned, in B-group vitamins and iron. In 1956 the British government, in releasing the milling and baking industry from the controls imposed in the 1939–45 war, stipulated the minimum contents of thiamine, nicotinic acid, calcium and iron in flour of whatever extraction rate the industry chose, deficits being added as pure chemicals (presumably the thiamine and nicotonic acid are made from the discarded part of the wheat grain!). Calcium is added as calcium carbonate, the chief component of chalk and limestone, iron as finely divided metallic iron or ferric ammonium citrate, neither of which is absorbed from the gut! It is now doubtful whether, apart from the uselessness of the iron added, any of the other three additives are needed in British food of the 1970s, for they are present in abundance in other foods. Furthermore, adding only thiamine and nicotinic acid of the B group of vitamins, does not help to replace the quantity of several others of the group that are removed in preparing 70% extraction flour. For these nutritional reasons, I would favour the use of a high extraction flour.

There is one possible disadvantage to this, however. This is in the phytic acid content of 100% extraction flour which reduces calcium and iron absorption. The evidence on the significance of this is conflicting. Rickets due to deficient calcium absorption undoubtedly occurred among Irish children in 1940 when only 100% extraction flour was allowed, and in experimental animals, as was reported at about the same time. The percentage of calcium in bread that is absorbed was found to be far higher in white or 'dephytinised' brown bread than in untreated brown bread in 1942. But wheat flour also contains a phytic acid destroying enzyme, *phytase*. The leavening process in bread making may produce the right conditions for phytase to act. Thus the phytic acid of 100% flour can be destroyed and so not hinder calcium or iron absorption. (Phytic acid in other foods is not so destroyed.)

Bread is the chief form in which wheat flour is eaten. Because of the added water, all the components of the wheat are present in somewhat reduced amounts when compared with the original flour, as is seen in Table 6.7. Flour is mixed with water to form a 'workable' dough. To this is added a small amount of sugar, fat and a growing yeast preparation. The yeast attacks the sugar, producing carbon dioxide. This causes the leavening or rising of the dough mixture, and it will only happen if the temperature is high enough (25°C or 77°F) and the yeast actively growing. One of the wheat proteins, *gluten*, makes the risen dough so firm that it will keep its shape until it has been placed in an oven at 230°C (425°F) and baked. This, by a combination of partial drying out of the dough and alteration of the proteins (heat coagulation), permanently stabilises the dough so that once it has risen and been cooked it retains its light spongy texture. The cooking process effectively sterilises the bread, killing the yeast and any other microorganisms that might have been present, and if kept in a cool and dry place a well-made wholemeal loaf remains palatable for several days. Palatability is restored to stale bread by reheating it. The term 'biscuit' originally derived from the French, and meaning twice-cooked was first applied to bread treated in this way (see Alfred Duggan's *Knight with Armour*, an imaginative re-creation of the first Crusade).

Table 6.7 Composition of typical breads (per 100g).

	Protein g	Fat g	Carbohydrate g	Calcium mg	Iron mg	Thiamine mg	Energy MJ
100% Wholemeal	8.2	2.0	47.1	26.0	2.88	0.20	0.96
90% Wholemeal	8.7	2.1	49.9	95.0	2.44	0.21	1.00
70% White bread	8.0	1.4	51.7	91.0	1.82	0.18	1.00

Biscuits, cakes, currant buns etc. are nowadays made from wheat flour, sugar and fat and dried fruits. Yeast may or may not be used to cause the dough mixture to rise. They owe their energy content partly to the wheat flour and partly to the other added materials. The thiamine content of these is unknown, but the other components are shown in Table 6.8. Some biscuits are very rich energy sources, because of their added fat or carbohydrate content.

Some *breakfast cereals* are made from wheat. They are a more expensive

Table 6.8 Composition of biscuits, cakes etc. (per 100g).

	Protein g	Fat g	Carbohydrate g	Calcium mg	Iron mg	Energy MJ
Digestive biscuits	9.6	20.5	66.0	111	2.01	2.02
Plain biscuits	7.4	13.2	75.3	126	1.78	1.81
Sweet biscuits	5.5	30.7	66.5	83	1.20	2.32
Fruit cake	6.1	18.0	60.2	194	1.29	1.75
Currant buns	7.4	7.6	54.5	90	2.49	1.28

way than is bread of obtaining the same weight of energy-providing material, though the milk commonly eaten with these preparations provides a useful protein additive. The composition of some wheat-derived and other breakfast cereals is given in Table 6.9. The thiamine and nicotinic acid are added to these products during their preparation.

Table 6.9 The composition of some breakfast cereals (per 100g).

	Protein g	Fat g	Carbo-hydrate g	Calcium mg	Iron mg	Thiamine mg	Nicotinic acid mg	Energy MJ
All Bran	12.6	4.5	58.0	82.1	10.80	1.1	15.9	1.30
Puffed Wheat	13.9	2.0	75.3	35.3	3.29	1.1	15.9	1.50
Shredded Wheat	9.7	2.8	79.0	34.8	4.48	1.1	15.9	1.51
Cornflakes	6.6	0.8	88.2	7.4	2.80	1.1	15.9	1.53
Oatmeal porridge (made with water)	1.4	0.9	8.2	6.3	0.47	0.1	0.1	0.19
Rice Krispies	5.7	1.1	85.1	6.1	0.72	1.1	15.9	1.46

Triticum durum flour is used for making pasta. When dried and marketed this is comparable in composition to the original flour, though a considerable loss of thiamine occurs in making pasta. When cooked, a pasta will absorb twice its weight of water, so its energy content falls from 1.5 MJ/100 g as bought to 0.47 MJ/100 g when ready to eat.

Finally, people in and from Northern India make chapattis from wheat flour. The dough is made by adding water, salt and a little fat. It is rolled flat and cooked on a flat iron plate. The energy value will depend upon the amount of added fat and the final water content of the cooked product.

Rice

What wheat is to Europe and North America, rice is to the inhabitants of South and East Asia. It needs a warm and moist climate for its growth, but as in wheat cultivation, man has extended the original range and productivity of rice by selective breeding. Again, as with wheat, it has always been fashionable to remove the outer layers of the rice grain, and to eat only the pure white endosperm. This process is known as polishing. It removes over 90% of the thiamine and much of the protein (less anyway than in wheat). We normally use rice as polished whole grains which are boiled and washed in fresh boiling water before being eaten. The protein, carbohydrate and energy values of the raw and boiled polished grains are shown in Table 6.10. It should be noted that much of the thiamine that was retained in the raw polished grain (by *parboiling* before polishing) may be lost in the water used for cooking the grain. In cooking, rice takes up 2 parts of water for every part of solid material, so cooked rice is a bulky food, compared with, say, the cooking of wheat flour to make bread. Careful cooking of brown rice, by allowing the water to almost completely evaporate when the grain is fully cooked, enhances both the nutritional quality and the flavour of the product. Fried rice will have a higher energy content than boiled rice, owing to the fat that remains adherent to the grains.

Table 6.10 Composition of raw and cooked rice (per 100g).

	Protein	Fat	Carbo-hydrate	Calcium	Iron	Thiamine	Nicotinic acid	Energy
	g	g	g	mg	mg	mg	mg	MJ
Polished, raw	6.2	1.0	86.8	3.7	0.45	0.08	1.5	1.50
Polished, cooked	2.1	0.3	29.6	1.3	0.16	0.01	0.3	0.51

Maize

This originated in the more arid southern parts of North America and was introduced to Europe, Africa and Asia in the sixteenth and subsequent centuries. It can be ground to a fine flour, or cooked as whole grains. The composition of maize flour is given in Table 6.11, together with that of some preparations derived from it. Cornflour is the endosperm starch from which the more soluble protein has been washed away. Whole grain maize is cooked as a porridge in Africa and as tortillas in Mexico. The flour will not make leavened bread on its own, but can readily be mixed with wheat flour in bread-making. In the cooking process the energy content of the final product will depend on its water content. More will be said about maize in Chapters 8 and 9, concerning its protein and vitamin content.

Table 6.11 Composition of maize flour and some products (per 100g).

	Protein	Fat	Carbo-hydrate	Calcium	Iron	Thiamine	Nicotinic acid	Energy
	g	g	g	mg	mg	mg	mg	MJ
Maize flour	7.1	1.3	77.5	?	?	?	?	1.50
Cornflakes	6.6	0.8	88.2	7.4	2.8	1.1	15.9	1.53
Cornflour and custard powder	0.5	0.7	92.0	15.2	1.4	trace	trace	1.47

Some varieties of maize contain appreciable amounts of sugar and are known as *sweet corn*. This may be eaten on the cob or after the whole grains have been removed. It is commonly served with butter, which enhances its energy value as a food.

Oats

This cereal is exceptional in that its flour contains 9% of fat, and its energy value is 1.7 MJ/100 g (wheat flour is 1.4–1.5 MJ). However it cannot form a leavened bread and is little used now for human consumption, except as porridge, in which, as seen in Table 6.9, it has an energy value of 0.19 MJ/100 g about one fifth that of bread.

Barley

This is now used for animal feeds, and for beer making, though it was formerly used for human consumption, the flour being mixed with wheat flour. Whole grains, *pearl barley*, are occasionally used in stews. Their energy value, when dry, is about 1.5 MJ/100 g, since they are about 84% carbohydrate.

Rye

Like wheat, rye has been used extensively as the basis for bread-making, though rye flour contains little gluten, and therefore will not make a leavened bread on its own. It is commonly mixed with wheat. Pure rye flour has a composition similar to wheat, except that the protein content is lower, and 30–40% of the protein are not digested or absorbed in the human gut.

Rye will grow and ripen in climates too cool and damp for wheat, though the dampness may favour the growth of *ergot*, a fungus which produces a series of poisonous alkaloids. 'Saint Anthony's Fire' is the disease resulting from these compounds. Widespread in the Middle Ages, ergot poisoning was almost certainly the cause of an outbreak that affected a town in Southern France in 1954. The drug LSD, taken by the foolhardy for its psychotropic effects, is an ergot derivative and, in my opinion, as dangerous as any of these alkaloids. They have the peculiar property of remaining attached to nerve cells and affecting their function for many weeks after being ingested.

The pulses

These are the seeds of many of the leguminous plants, now called Fabaceae by the botanists. All must be mixed with water for cooking. When cooked, pulses swell to about $2\frac{1}{2}$ or 3 times their dry bulk with a comparable change in composition and energy value. Table 6.12 gives this composition when dry. Their high protein content is noted here in passing. It will be considered further in Chapter 8. Soya bean flour owes its high energy content to its fat, unlike the other pulse products which have between 45 and 60% carbohydrate. As was seen in Table 6.2, the fat of soya bean and ground nut contains a considerable amount of the polyunsaturated fatty acid fats. Some pulses are now coming to attention because they contain significant amounts of non-digestible polysaccharide substances ('fibre') which may have the same beneficial effects described for wheat bran on page 59 of this chapter.

Table 6.12 Composition of some raw dried pulses (per 100g).

	Protein	Fat	Carbo-hydrate	Calcium	Iron	Thiamine	Nicotinic acid	Energy
	g	g	g	mg	mg	mg	mg	MJ
Haricot beans	21.4	trace	45.5	180	6.65	0.45	2.5	1.07
Lentils	23.8	trace	53.2	39	7.62	0.50	2.5	1.23
Split peas	22.1	trace	56.6	33	5.40	0.70	3.2	1.26
Soya bean flour	40.3	23.5	13.3	208	6.93	0.75	2.0	1.81
Ground nuts (roasted)	28.1	4.9	8.6	61	2.04	0.23	16.0	2.51

Root vegetables

Cassava (tapioca) is prepared from the roots of a tropical shrub, *Manihot utilissima*. This contains 50–75% water, less than 1% protein, and the remainder mostly starch. The starch has to be separated from a poisonous cyanide-containing compound before it can be eaten. Arrowroot is another starch prepared from plant roots. It contains only 0.4% protein and 94% available carbohydrate. The root vegetables in common use, such as beet-root, carrots, leeks, onions, parsnips, swedes and turnips contain between 4 and 11% starch and thus have an energy value of 0.08–0.22 MJ/100 g.

Tubers and stems

Though many tubers develop below the surface of the ground, they are botanically stems and properly should be called 'underground stems' to distinguish them from true roots.

Potatoes

Again, a plant obtained from America after the European discoveries, this has become of great importance in nutrition throughout the temperate world and has affected the whole development of Ireland and the USA for over a century. Under ideal conditions an acre of ground can produce a potato crop containing over three times as much usable energy as the same ground growing wheat or other grain crops. All this energy content, moreover, is directly available to Man, if he can be induced or forced to eat it! Potatoes are prepared in various ways and the final composition and energy values are shown in Table 6.13. In mashing, roasting and frying, fat is added and in the latter two cooking processes, and in baking, water loss also leads to an enhancement of the energy value of potatoes.

Other tubers

Yams, sweet potato and taro are all grown in various tropical and sub-tropical countries. Their compositions and energy values are similar to potatoes. *Sago* is an almost pure starch prepared from the pith of the sago palm. The dry preparation, containing 94% starch, has an energy value of 1.48 MJ/100 g. In cooking, like many other materials, sago grains swell up

Table 6.13 The composition of potatoes, raw and variously cooked (per 100g).

	Protein	Fat	Carbo-hydrate	Calcium	Iron	Thiamine	Nicotinic acid	Energy
	g	g	g	mg	mg	mg	mg	MJ
Old, raw	2.1	trace	20.8	7.7	0.75	0.11	1.2	0.36
Old, boiled (peeled)	1.4	trace	19.7	4.3	0.48	0.08	0.8	0.34
Old, mashed	1.5	5.0	18.0	11.7	0.45	?	?	0.50
Old, baked	2.5	trace	25.0	9.2	0.90	0.10	1.2	0.44
Old, roast	2.8	1.0	27.3	10.1	0.99	0.10	1.2	0.52
Old, chips	3.8	9.0	37.3	13.8	1.35	0.10	1.2	1.00
New, boiled	1.6	trace	18.3	5.0	0.46	0.08	0.8	0.31

to about 3 times their dry size with a corresponding reduction in energy value.

7
Proteins and nutrition

The chemistry of amino acids and how they link together to form proteins has already been described in Chapter 3. In human nutrition (but not that of some other mammals) the amine (NH_2) group must already be incorporated into the amino acids, as must the side chains of 8 of the 20 amino acids. These 8 are therefore called the *essential* amino acids. The protein nutritional requirements for man are thus a sufficient total amino acid intake to meet the demands of growth and daily maintenance, together with sufficient of the essential amino acids for growth, maintenance and some metabolic needs.

The amino acids from the digested food proteins enter a common metabolic pool in blood and other body fluids. Individual body cells take from this pool those amino acids that they require for their metabolic needs: growth, replacement and enzyme formation etc. In addition, some of the protein in liver cells and up to half that in skeletal muscle can be regarded as a protein store, for these proteins may be broken down to their constituent amino acids which then enter the metabolic pool. Some amino acids have very specific synthetic functions in the body and, if not present in the food, can be obtained in this way from liver and muscle protein. Surpluses of other (usually non-essential) amino acids may then accumulate in the pool. These may be oxidised by the common metabolic pathways leading to energy transfer (indeed, as has already been seen in Chapter 5, oxidation is the ultimate fate of the bulk of food protein and it yields as much energy as carbohydrate oxidation). The amine group, however, cannot be oxidised, it is lost to the body in the urine as urea.

Urea is the principal waste product of protein metabolism in the body. The other minor nitrogen-containing waste products are also excreted in the urine, so a determination of daily urea or urinary nitrogen amounts gives a good indication of the rate of protein catabolism in the body, though it cannot distinguish between the breakdown of food and of body proteins (exogenous or endogenous protein catabolism respectively).

It is the use of these concepts of the common amino acid pool, and the entry into it of both food and body proteins, together with measurements of urea or urinary nitrogen and of growth rates, that has enabled us to determine how much protein, and how much of each individual essential amino acid is needed in our food. Most of the necessarily difficult and lengthy experiments have been performed on small laboratory animals, but sufficient confirmation has been obtained in human subjects to enable guidelines to be drawn up for our nutrition.

Minimal protein needs

If a person is maintained on a protein-free diet, he will perforce utilise body (liver and skeletal muscle) proteins as a source of the amino acids needed for more urgent metabolic processes. In these circumstances such a person loses nitrogen equivalent to 22 g of protein.

Theoretically, if one knew the exact amino acid mix of this essential protein metabolism, and could find a protein with this same amino acid composition, then 22 g of such a protein in the food would replace the inevitable amino acid losses from the metabolic pool. This, in fact, is not possible. We do not know the exact amino acid mix and if we did it is most unlikely that it would be met in a single food protein, or food substance. Whatever protein, or protein-containing food, we add to the diet will contain some of the amino acids needed in the metabolic pool, and some surplus amino acids. The nitrogen from these will eventually appear in the urine. The experimental trick is to go on adding protein to the food until food protein supplies all the required amino acids for the common metabolic pool, and none need to be obtained from endogenous (liver and muscle) protein. Before this state has been reached, the nitrogen in the urine, coming partly from food and partly from body protein, will exceed the nitrogen in the food protein. When food protein supplies all the bodily needs, then nitrogen loss will equal nitrogen intake. This important state is called being in *nitrogen balance*. In different sets of experiments the smallest amount of food protein needed to achieve nitrogen balance has varied from 21 to 65 g of protein daily. We must now examine the daily requirements of essential amino acids in more detail, and then consider their distribution in various food proteins.

Essential amino acids

Though we talk of the 8 essential amino acids, isoleucine, leucine, lysine, methionine, phenylalanine, threonine, tryptophan and valine, we have to remember that histidine is also needed for growth in children, also that phenylalanine in the body is converted to tyrosine (which is also present in food proteins) and may itself have to be excluded from the diet in certain people with a metabolic disorder. Using the technique of determining nitrogen balance in people fed proteins of known amino acid composition, research workers have arrived at estimates of the amount of each essential amino acid needed per person (adult or infant) per day. For adults these vary from 250 mg for tryptophan to 1 g for leucine, methionine and phenylalanine (or tyrosine). The values have also been determined per kg of body weight and range from 3.5 to 14 mg/kg/day. Corresponding values for infants are 17–160 mg/kg/day, and 28 mg/kg of histidine is also needed each day in infants. The much higher values for infants are a reflection of their greater metabolic rate and their growth rate.

Obviously, the total daily protein intake will be determined by these requirements of essential amino acids, and the exact amount of protein needed will depend upon the amino acid composition of the food proteins. Without giving numerical scores to different foods' proteins, I would like here to say simply that *animal proteins more nearly match, in amino acid composition, the metabolic needs of humans*, that different vegetable proteins have small amounts of different essential amino acids, but that a *careful combination of different vegetable materials may provide as good a dietary intake of amino acids as one containing meat or cheese.*

I will go into this last point in more detail. Wheat endosperm protein, in common with most grain proteins, has little lysine, but wheat germ protein has as much as milk and eggs. Beans also are rich in lysine and endeavours in the early 1970s have produced a high lysine containing maize variety. Beans, though, have one-third the methionine content of wheat and one-fifth that of meat. By mixing beans with wheat or rice (the Mexican dish of chile con carne with rice, for instance), one achieves a reasonable mixture of all the essential amino acids. It is, of course, when a single vegetable foodstuff, be it wheat, potatoes, rice or other energy-providing food, becomes the major part of the total food intake, that shortages of particular amino acids may occur.

The daily optimal protein intake

While many authorities used to put this at or above 100 g/day for the adult, nitrogen balance has been obtained at values ranging from 21 g to 65 g/day. A useful standard would be to accept 1 g/kg body weight/day (since adult men weigh, on average, 70 kg). This is the figure accepted by both FAO and the USA National Research Council. The latter authority states that pregnant and nursing mothers should receive 1.5 g/kg/day and 1.8 g/kg/day respectively. It is little more than a rule-of-thumb sort of guideline, but it is also generally recommended that 10% of the total energy value of the daily food intake should be protein and that half of this should be animal origin, i.e. the meat, fish, milk, cheese or eggs in the daily diet should contain not less than 35 g protein. It is a simple enough exercise, using the food tables to determine the protein intake of a specimen diet. I have already described such a diet (p. 40) and I can here show how much protein this supplies. For each component the protein content per 100 g is found from food tables and multiplied by the weight of that food, as in Table 7.1. Bread contains 8 g protein/100 g, so 250 g bread contains $2.5 \times 8 = 20$ g protein. It will be seen from this example that the total protein intake was 94.05 g, of which 22.65 g was of vegetable origin while 71.4 g came from animal sources. This diet is clearly one containing more meat, eggs, milk and cheese than is necessary. It reflects, perhaps, the choice of a relatively wealthy and self-indulgent person! Another useful exercise would be to determine how much meat, bread, or even potatoes would have to be eaten to satisfy daily protein needs if one were to accept the 70 g/day standard, regardless of its source. It works out at 5 kg of potatoes (which would supply 16 MJ of energy!). Table 7.2 shows how much of the various animal foods are needed to give the recommended daily protein intake.

Table 7.1 The protein content of a specimen diet

	Amount eaten g or ml/day	Protein contents g/100g	Protein provided g or ml/day
Bread	250g	8	20
Milk	500ml	3.4	17
Bacon	75g	14	10.5
Egg	50g	12	6
Meat	125g	20	25
Cheese	50g	25.4	12.7
Butter	50g	0.4	0.2
Potatoes	100g	1.4	1.4
Cabbage	100g	1.1	1.1
Jam	25g	0.6	0.15
Sugar	50g	nil	nil
Total			94.05

Table 7.2 The amount of various foods supplying 35g of animal protein.

		As purchased	Ready to eat
Cheese (Cheddar)	(g)	138	138
Milk	(l)	1.08	1.08
Eggs	(g)	260 (5 size 2)	260
Cod	(g)	255	170
Sole	(g)	270	175
Herring	(g)	210	160
Bacon	(g)	270	145
Shin Beef	(g)	180	115
Leg Pork	(g)	160	140
Liver	(g)	210	120
Chicken	(g)	150	120

The edible portions of cooked fish and meat which give 35 g are smaller than the amounts 'as purchased'. This is because of the wastage before cooking and the water lost during cooking.

The practical advantage of such a list is that one can readily see whether a diet contains enough animal protein. Thus 0.5 l of milk contains half the daily requirement, 125 g of beef contains over this amount, 50 g of cheese about one-third of the amount and so on. The specimen diet of Table 7.1 contains twice the required amount of animal protein, as already noted.

Whatever the agreed daily optimum may be, actual protein intake is frequently determined by economic necessity, or by personal and social factors. The poor in many parts of the world may eat less than 50 g/day, as may some as a result of their religious or personal beliefs. In the UK and many other wealthy countries, people choose (as in the example quoted above) to eat more than the optimum. The Masai and the Eskimo eat 200–300 g/day. Does any harm result from the low and the high protein intake of some people?

Individual intakes of total and animal protein

When we look at the actual protein intakes of men, women and children, determined from individual diet surveys we find that, while the average figure compares favourably with the recommended figure, the individual departures are great.

Thus, in the example in Table 7.1, the total daily protein intake was 94 g, of which 71 g came from animal sources. In one survey, on middle-class households only, one man had an animal protein intake less than 35 g, the average was 67 g and one person consumed 120 g. In the women, the average was 46 g and the range 9–64 g. Total protein amounts in both men and women were similarly varied.

On turning to children and adolescents (in whom the protein requirements are more critical than for adults, except for pregnant and nursing mothers and those recovering from illness, injury or operation) we do find a close similarity between the average intakes and the estimated needs. Figure 7.1 shows how close is this agreement. Once again one must remember that the averages conceal a considerable variation and that in any one age group we may find one child eating twice as much protein as another of the same age.

How much, for both children and adults, of the total protein should be of animal origin, remains unsettled. The rule-of-thumb guide states that it should be not less than half the total protein. But this guide is concerned with the intake of essential amino acids, and we now have the exact amino acid composition of the proteins of many different foodstuffs, and some reasonable estimates of the daily requirement of each essential amino acid. One could, therefore replace a rule-of-thumb rule with a host of exact prescriptions, or find, for example, that a judicious mixture of wheat, rice or maize with beans or pulses is quite as good as meat, milk and eggs. To replace one empirical rule with another, vegetable proteins of mixed origin (not just cereals) are as good as animal proteins, and if you add to that 0.5 l of milk you cannot go far wrong (so long as lactose intolerance does not preclude milk).

Could our total intake of protein be too high?

Figures as high as some in the previous two sections have been criticised as being in excess of needs, and workers have referred to 'primitive people' or 'peasants' who live to a ripe old age on diets containing far less protein. They fail to recognise the logical flaws—many people on a high protein also live to old age and in the same state of health—and many of the primitives or peasants died young. Then there is a belief that a high protein diet overworks the kidneys, leads to cancer or 'auto-intoxication', due to the production of tyramine and histamine, both of which are poisonous, from tyrosine and histidine (two amino acids) in the colon. But no one has ever shown that Eskimos or Masai, whose diet is largely protein, have a greater incidence of kidney disease. Why should we, furthermore, show such solicitude for the

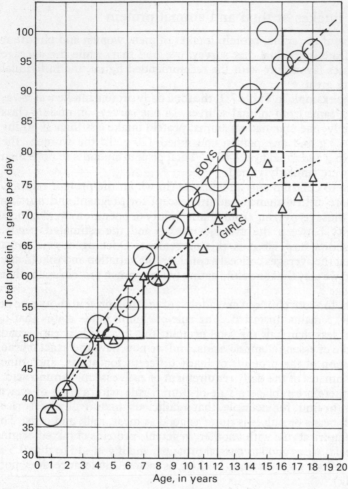

Fig. 7.1 Graph of actual intakes of protein by 1000 English middle-class boys and girls compared with American estimated needs.

Circles represent boys; triangles, girls. Smoothed curves have been drawn freehand through the actual figures for boys and girls to suggest what the intakes would have been if the number of observations had been indefinitely increased. The firm stepped line represents American estimates for boys and girls till 13 and thereafter that of boys only. From 13 the estimates for girls are shown in dashes.

Except that the boys and girls take rather more than the American estimates in the earlier years there is an astonishingly close agreement.

kidneys? They are concerned far more with maintaining the body's salt and water balances than with excreting the nitrogenous end-products of protein metabolism. Likewise, there is no greater incidence of cancer in high protein eaters, and the myth of auto-intoxication was disproved many years ago. Finally, may I once again remind you that the human race evolved as a meat-eating species, and it is only pressure of numbers that has driven us to a more vegetarian diet.

However one can argue that, because some people *can* live in excellent health on as little as 40 g protein a day, and because the cost of producing the foods of such a diet—in cash and acreage of land—is less than that of producing a high-protein diet, the aim of all nutritionists should be to wean people onto a minimal and mainly vegetable protein diet. In any case the gap between the low protein intake of many healthy people and the higher internationally agreed figures should make any scientist pause and think again!

Possible advantages of a high protein diet

First, the fact that the species evolved as a meat-eating species means that we are adapted to meat-eating. For some millions of years our human and sub-human ancestors ate meat, and it is only in the last 10 000 years that we have turned our attention to plant foods. Our metabolic machinery has not had time to change its nature.

When a person switches to a low protein diet, the output of nitrogen in the urine does not fall immediately to a comparable level. It takes some days for the metabolic processes to adjust to the change. Similarly, when he reverts to a high protein diet, considerable retention of nitrogen occurs, with a consequent lag in urinary nitrogen loss behind intake, before he once again achieves a nitrogen balance state.

Ever since the production of radioactively labelled amino acids and their quantitative estimation became available, the dynamic nature of proteins in body cells has been appreciated. Proteins are constantly being broken down and renewed. Many of the non-essential amino acids are freely interchangeable with other substances in the body and all amino acids, essential and non-essential, can be considered as existing in a 'pool', in blood and tissue fluids. This amino acid pool is normally replenished by dietary proteins. It *can* be maintained by skeletal muscle or liver protein. It is continually losing all amino acids into new protein formation, and essential amino acids into various metabolic pathways. Most amino acids, with the particular exception of lysine, can interchange amine groups with other similar but amine-free compounds. The amine groups of surplus, usually non-essential amino acids are converted to urea and lost to the body in the urine. This rapid, extensive and continuous interchange between amino acids of the pool and those of tissue proteins is a mark of life. It must sink to a lower level as the pool is reduced in size, as happens when a low protein diet is taken. We must ask whether there is any evidence that producing a low level of tissue protein metabolism is either beneficial or harmful. While we know that some people *can* carry on with a low level of this activity, others cannot and that 'in order to be sure we have enough we must have too much'. Furthermore after illness, injury or operations there may be an extra demand for methionine. If the diet does not contain an excess of this amino acid, tissue (skeletal muscle) protein will be broken down to obtain the methionine needed to restore bodily function. The importance of lysine can similarly be seen. Human tissues (including skeletal muscle) contain 6.6% lysine. In the young, in pregnant and nursing mothers, convalescents and in athletes, the dietary intake of lysine is important. There is 8.2% lysine in the caseinogen (the main protein) of milk and over 6% in meat and egg proteins, while there is only 2.5% in wheat endosperm protein. Again, the advantages of a high protein—particularly animal protein—diet in these states should be clear.

The disadvantages of a low protein diet

A low protein intake affects growth adversely in embryo, infant, child or adolescent. In infants growth of the brain is permanently impaired with, possibly, a limitation also of intellectual performance. Throughout the growing period in childhood and adolescence growth will be restricted by protein deficiency. Short periods of such restriction do no harm, for the child can subsequently catch up the deficit, when he once again receives an adequate diet. Longer periods of restriction result in permanent reduction in size. Bone growth and development is similarly affected, the characteristic milestones being achieved later than normal.

Replacement, which is simply growth in a different sense, is also affected. The tissue which replaces itself most rapidly is the epithelial lining of the intestine. The life of the individual cells is about 3 days. In addition, these cells are constantly producing protein enzymes, as are the cells of stomach and pancreas. For these reasons, protein deficiency may produce diarrhoea and consequent loss of water, salts etc. and further exacerbate the nutritional deficiency. The liver is affected and fat droplets appear on its cells (methionine lack may be the most important factor here). The liver also makes the chief protein, albumin, of blood plasma. Albumin is the 'carrier' for many of the materials normally transported between the various tissues of the body. It also 'holds', by osmotic attraction, the water of the blood plasma in the circulation. If the albumin concentration is low, water leaks from the blood into the tissue fluids and oedema develops. Haemoglobin formation is reduced, resulting in anaemia.

Finally, skeletal muscle protein can be used in an attempt to maintain essential amino acid levels, and muscle weakness and wasting develops in all cases of excessively low protein diets.

Illnesses, particularly infectious ones, increase the body's needs for protein, for white blood cell formation and for the production of antibodies. A barely adequate diet becomes frankly inadequate when these extra demands are made, and as the defence against the illness is reduced, so it is increased in severity and duration.

Severe protein deficiency seen when infants in some tropical countries are first weaned from the breast onto protein-poor cereal foods, is known as kwashiorkor, in which the gastro-intestinal liver and blood disorders described above are prominent.

Timing of protein in meals

Since most of the amino acids can have their amine groups removed and then be oxidised by the common metabolic paths for all foodstuffs, it is obviously essential to avoid an undue separation of the major foodstuffs between meals. At one time, a regimen known as the Hay diet was advocated. In this, the taking of carbohydrate and protein in the same meal was forbidden. Thus potatoes with meat, or bread and cheese were prohibited. All the available amino acids from a meat-only meal that could be converted to glucose would be so converted, for the liver has an overriding commitment to maintain an adequate glucose level in the blood. It is therefore advisable, as the great majority of us have always done, to combine protein and carbohydrate in the same meals, eating cheese *and* bread, meat *and* potatoes, fish *and* chips. Dietary regimes should be based on knowledge, not fancy, as was the Hay diet.

Estimation of protein intake

In principle, this is very similar to the estimation of the energy intake. One can directly measure the nitrogen output (urea, uric acid and other compounds in the urine) which must be equal to the nitrogen intake, on average and provided the person is in nitrogen balance. Since 100 g of protein contains 16 g of nitrogen, the urinary nitrogen $\times$ 100/16 (i.e. urinary nitrogen $\times$ 6.25) gives the quantity of protein from which the urinary nitrogen is derived. The factor of 6.25 is the average for all food proteins. For cereal proteins it is 5.7 and for milk protein 6.28. Additional protein, equivalent to 1 g nitrogen, is lost by shedding of skin and in the faeces from shed epithelial cells.

The second method, measuring intake, is done by dietary survey methods, calculating from food composition tables the amount of protein consumed in the food. About 10% of the food protein (less for meat, fish or milk, more for some plant proteins) is not absorbed by the gut, so protein intake values are usually higher than the simultaneously calculated protein equivalent of urinary nitrogen excretion and the 1 g N allowed for other losses.

8

Protein-containing foods

Meat, poultry and offal

By meat one means, of course, the muscle tissue of mammals and birds, the great bulk of the edible material of these organisms. Meat was probably the main component of the diet of our ancestors, until agriculture took the place of hunting as our means of obtaining food, about 10 000 years ago. Meat remains the food we turn to by choice. When times are good we buy and eat more meat. When times are hard, it is the expensive meat we give up first, hoping for the return of better times when we will once again have unlimited meat. Englishmen are believed to need roast beef, and the American dream includes a chicken in every pot.

Upon this meat worship we should turn a sceptical and scientific eye. In its favour, one must note that the amino acid composition is most near to that of our body proteins (being largely muscle). Meats are good sources also of iron, of nicotinic acid, riboflavine and thiamine (especially in pork and bacon). Many meats contain appreciable amounts of fat, so their energy content is high. Meat is palatable, it is readily digested and the amino acids almost fully absorbed.

Against meat the sole argument is the economic one. It takes many kilograms of foodstuff (some of it perhaps edible for ourselves) and much time and effort to produce one kilogram of edible meat. Our desire for meat has led to over-stocking of large areas of land, and consequently to soil damage and destruction. If your meat could be solely obtained from animals that only ate materials we cannot live on ourselves this argument would have less value. Grass fed cattle, and sheep and pigs fed on nuts, roots and any vegetables they can find make better sense than giving grain to cattle or fish meal to the pigs.

The palatability of meat depends largely upon its tenderness. This is dependent partly upon cooking methods, but also upon the amount of connective tissue present in it and the length of time after death of the animal that it is cooked. Shortly after any animal dies, its muscles go into *rigor mortis*. This lasts for several hours and meat cooked in this state is sure to be tough. The meat must be 'hung' until rigor mortis has passed off. During the rigor mortis phase, furthermore, the meat becomes acidic, since lactic acid is formed from the glycogen present in the muscle tissue. Lactic acid helps to break down connective tissue, so its presence also tenderises the meat. Vinegar (acetic acid) will do the same, and the best artificial meat tenderising agent will contain enzymes that split the collagen of connective tissue.

The fat of meat, which contributes so largely to its energy content, is found with the connective tissues, between the muscles. In different species of animals, and in different joints cut from the same animal, the amount of fat is very variable. Chicken and turkey are largely free of fat, but goose and duck are rich in fat. Beef is rich but venison is poor, and so is veal. Shoulder and chops of lamb contain much more fat than the leg joint from the same beast. Table 8.1 gives the composition of some meats. Although all muscle contains 1–3% of glycogen during life, most, if not all of this is converted to lactic acid in hanging. The food tables show all meats (except liver) as being carbohydrate-free.

Offals (which means 'off fall') are also good meat sources of protein, though their lower fat content gives them a lower energy value. The protein is as valuable as the meat protein and, as Table 8.2 shows, different offals may contribute in a marked way to our intake of various vitamins, and of iron and calcium. The problems are those of acceptability and palatability, and various ways have been found to encourage us to eat such materials as blood or the tough and strongly flavoured pig's liver (black pudding and faggots).

Meat is difficult to preserve. Salting and drying, with or without wood-smoke, have been used for many centuries. Nowadays it is the pig that is so treated to produce bacon and ham. While the protein and fat will be excellently preserved by such measures there is some loss of thiamine, and nicotinic acid but none of riboflavine. Many meats are now preserved in cans, of which corned beef is the traditional example. Losses of nicotinic acid are less than in bacon production, but the thiamine is almost totally lost. Since much water is removed in making corned beef, its protein content is higher than that of fresh beef. The fat content can be adjusted at the will of the manufacturer to suit palatability. It may well be less than that of a joint of fresh beef. Table 8.3 gives the composition of some preserved meats. It should be compared with Table 8.1 to see how the preservation has affected the product's composition.

Soups, meat stock and meat extracts

There is an old belief that since the flavours of meat can readily be extracted into stock etc., which may then be used to make soups, the nutritional value also is extracted. This is of course, a mistaken belief. Neither the bulk of the protein nor the fat is present in these extracts. Soup made from meat derives its value almost entirely from other substances added in its preparation. These include flour and fat in the making of a thick soup, or milk, pasta, peas or potatoes added to various special soups.

Gelatin is also extracted from meat. It is obtained from collagen, the chief component of connective tissue, by boiling. Although gelatin is rich in histidine (an essential amino acid for the young), the jellies made from it are so diluted that the amount of this amino acid obtained by eating jelly is negligible.

Table 8.1 Composition of typical meats, after cooking (per 100g).

	Protein g	Fat g	Calcium mg	Iron mg	Thiamine mg	Riboflavine mg	Nicotinic acid mg	Energy MJ
Beef (roast)	24.2	23.8	5.9	4.4	0.05	0.22	5.0	1.34
Veal (roast)	30.5	11.5	14.3	2.5	0.06	0.27	7.0	0.97
Lamb (leg roast)	25.0	20.4	4.3	4.3	0.10	0.25	4.5	1.22
Pork (leg roast)	24.6	23.2	5.2	1.7	0.80	0.20	5.0	1.32
Chicken (on bone roast)	16.0	3.9	7.8	1.4	0.03	0.07	3.3	0.43
Chicken (meat only roast)	29.6	7.3	14.5	2.6	0.05	0.13	6.0	0.79
Duck (on bone, roast)	12.3	12.8	10.2	3.1	?	?	?	0.71
Duck (meat only, roast)	22.8	23.6	19.0	5.8	?	?	?	1.31

Table 8.2 Composition of some meat offals after cooking (per 100g).

	Protein g	Fat g	Carbohydrate g	Calcium mg	Iron mg	Retinol µg	Thiamine mg	Ascorbic acid mg	Energy MJ
Heart (lamb, roast)	25.0	14.7	nil	9.5	8.1	60	0.20	nil	1.00
Kidney (lamb, fried)	28.0	9.1	nil	16.6	14.5	300	?	6	0.83
Liver (calf, fried)	29.0	14.5	2.4	8.8	21.7	6000	0.30	20	1.10
Tripe (stewed)	18.0	3.0	nil	127.0	1.6	?	?	?	0.43

Table 8.3 Composition of preserved meats.

	Protein g	Fat g	Calcium mg	Iron mg	Thiamine mg	Riboflavine mg	Nicotinic acid mg	Energy MJ
Corned beef	22.3	15.0	12.8	9.8	trace	0.20	3.5	0.97
Boiled ham	16.3	39.6	12.7	2.5	0.50	0.20	3.5	1.82
Tinned 'luncheon meat'	11.4	29.0	17.5	1.1	0.40	0.20	3.5	1.40

Fish

The value of fish as a protein food in public estimation comes, for most of us, some way after meat, though in some more northern European countries it takes the place of meat, as it did on 'fast' days in earlier centuries of the Christian era. In other parts of the world nowadays, fish is a more readily available source of animal protein than are mammalian or avian meat or other products.

Both when purchased and when served there is a larger wastage with fish than with the other meats. There is also more water in fish than in meat, and less fat. The fat content, indeed, ranges from 0.5% for cod, haddock and whiting, to 8% for mackerel and herrings in the autumn, and to 14% for herrings for the rest of the year, sprats and salmon. Even this value is far exceeded by most of the meats already described. As a consequence of the watery nature of fish and its low fat content, the energy value of fish is lower than that of meat. Finally, fish is poorer than meat in both the amount and variety of flavouring substances, so a fish diet becomes monotonous. Many people do not like the special flavours of fish. Table 8.4 gives the composition of some typical fish. It should be noted that the fat fish also contain the fat soluble vitamins, retinol and cholecalciferol.

In spite of the various drawbacks to fish, in the period between 1945 and 1975 there was a great increase in the world-wide catch of fish. While much of this was for direct human consumption, much was converted into 'fish meal' and fed to animals which were themselves subsequently slaughtered so that we could eat the meat so formed. The production of 'fish fingers' prepared *en masse* in factories, has also changed our fish-eating habits, and perhaps increased the proportion of caught fish that is wasted so far as direct human consumption is concerned. One consequence of this activity has been the grave reduction of stocks of many kinds of fish in some of the richest sea-fishing areas in the world, and in the later 1970s we are going to have to accept that sea-fish hunting cannot proceed in a totally uncontrolled manner if we wish to continue reaping the benefit of what the open sea can produce for us. A rational policy at the production end from the open sea, 'farming' of both salt- and fresh-water fish and an efficient distribution service can all help to ensure that we make the maximal use of this source of animal protein.

Fish can be preserved both by drying and smoking and by canning. Drying and smoking reduce the water content and that of thiamine, but do not affect the fat-soluble vitamins. Canning does destroy some of these vitamins, but tinned sardines and salmon still remain good sources of both.

Crustacea (crabs, lobsters and prawns) and molluscs (snails, oysters, whelks and mussels etc.) are also sources of animal protein that some regard, not as a seldom-to-be-tasted luxury, but more as a part of daily life. The same should be said of fish roe. Indeed, when preparing an earlier edition (1971) of this book, herring soft roe was one of the cheapest forms of

Table 8.4 The composition of some fish (per 100g).

	Protein g	Fat g	Calcium mg	Iron mg	Retinol μg	Thiamine mg	Riboflavine mg	Cholecalciferol μg	Energy MJ
Cod (steamed)	14.6	0.7	11.8	0.4	trace	0.06	0.10	nil	0.28
Cod (fried in butter)	18.8	4.3	45.2	0.9	trace	0.06	0.10	nil	0.61
Halibut (steamed)	17.3	3.0	9.9	0.5	120	0.08	0.10	1.0	0.41
Plaice (steamed)	9.8	1.0	20.4	0.3	trace	0.06	0.10	nil	0.21
Sole (steamed)	10.6	0.8	68.0	0.4	trace	0.06	0.10	nil	0.21
Herring (baked)	15.5	11.8	53.5	1.5	45	0.03	0.30	22.5	0.73
Mackerel (fried)	14.6	8.3	20.7	0.9	45	0.09	0.50	17.5	0.57
Salmon (steamed)	15.5	10.5	23.4	0.6	90	0.10	0.10	12.5	0.67

Note 1. The values are for the fish as served, i.e. with skin and bones.
Note 2. The values for the vitamins are for raw fish.

animal protein that could regularly be bought in the Cardiff fish market. I hardly ever see it now (1977). Has it been converted to fish-meal and fed to cattle or pigs?

Milk and cheese

While the protein content of milk is given in the food tables as 3.7 g/100 g, there is some variation from source to source. Not all breeds of cow produce the same milk, and in different places at different times man has obtained milk also from the sheep, goat, donkey and horse (quite apart from his own mother!). Although milk is the obligatory source of protein for the young infant, it can remain an important source throughout life, partially or wholly replaced by other foods after weaning. Milk proteins are an excellent source of animal protein, though some infants do have some difficulty in digesting the protein of cow's milk unless it has been boiled before being fed to the infant. A few people are lacking the enzyme lactase from birth, and many cease to form this enzyme after weaning. The resultant failure to absorb the milk sugar, lactose, may lead to digestive disorder and a consequent intolerance of milk. For this reason a valuable source of animal protein is denied to such people.

Liquid milk is of course very bulky and, being a good food source for micro-organisms as well as man, is difficult to store. While various dried milk powder preparations are now being produced, the traditional way of preserving milk has been as cheese.

The chief protein of milk, caseinogen, is precipitated as curds of calcium caseinate with the aid of a digestive enzyme, *rennin*. This precipitate carries with it the fat of the milk, so only a small fraction of the protein, lactalbumin, and the lactose remains in the *whey*. After pressing out most of the remaining water, the resultant curd is mixed with some salt or smoked to aid preservation and allowed to 'mature'. Bacteria originally present when the curd was formed, or added by deliberate inoculation, remain active during the maturation of the cheese and, according to some, greatly enhance its flavour. The protein content of different cheeses varies from 10.8 to 37.6%, though most are between 22 and 26%. The fat content varies from 23 to 40%. Variations in both protein and fat will depend upon the source of the milk and the exact way in which the cheese is prepared from it. A trace of lactose remains in most cheeses.

Casein has not as high a biological value as whole-milk protein and cheese is believed by some to be indigestible. This last is a myth and cheese is a valuable source of animal protein. Why is not more cheese eaten today? Three hundred years ago, the food of the armies of the British Civil Wars was bread, cheese and beer. As wealth increased and home-produced and imported meat became available all the year round, our consumption of cheese fell, until it was relegated to the position of a savoury, taken at the end of the meal when one had already had enough to eat. A wide variety of both home-produced and imported cheeses are nowadays readily available at prices which, for both protein and energy, are better than those of carcase meat. The dietitian ought, then, to look for all ways of promoting the fuller use of cheese.

Eggs

The egg has long been prized for convenience and its culinary virtues, but as a source of animal protein (and for everything else of value in it), the egg is an expensive commodity. The white consists of proteins, ovoalbumim being the chief one, in water. The total protein is about 9% of the egg white, which is about 60% of the whole egg. The yolk occupies about 30% of the whole egg and is 16% protein and 30% fat. The yolk and white proteins are all of high biological value, and are readily digested when cooked. There is some doubt about the digestibility of raw egg proteins.

Vegetable proteins

Much has already been said about the proteins of the grains and the pulses in Chapter 5. If one has to rely on these foods as a major source of energy, then one inevitably consumes a considerable amount of protein also. To take an absurd extreme, 800 g of bread would contain enough energy to satisfy a person's basal needs. It also contains nearly 70 g of protein, which, if it contained enough of all the essential amino acids, would satisfy this person's protein needs also. However, as already described, the wheat proteins cannot supply all our amino acid needs, and we need a mixture of proteins from different sources to achieve this. Grains are most deficient in lysine, but pulses have nearly as much lysine as does meat.

Apart from these, all green vegetables contain 1–3% protein. In many cases this protein is of high biological value and would be a valuable addition to the protein supply if it were present in larger amounts. The more rapidly growing points of vegetables, such as sprouting broccoli, brussels sprouts and cauliflower have over 3% protein, and potatoes about 2%.

'Novel' protein sources

As just mentioned, many green vegetables suitable for human consumption contain up to 3% protein of high biological value. Many inedible leafy materials and grasses also contain similar proteins, which can be extracted and worked up into a palatable form of food. Other such artificial sources of protein include marine plankton (small and microscopic animals and plants that swim or float near the sea's surface), yeasts and fungi which grow on various simple or exotic media (including aviation fuel), converting inorganic nitrogen-containing compounds into protein which can then be extracted and prepared so that it is suitable for human consumption. One such 'novel' protein source that will probably become economically viable is the protein that can be recovered when micro-organisms grow on sewage sludge. This protein would *not* be used for humans, but could be fed to pigs or chickens, in which about a third would be converted into edible meat. It is likely that this protein will, by 1990, cost no more than the conventional protein feeds for these animals, some of which cannot be fed directly to man. For the other schemes being proposed nowadays, it is possible that the cost in energy equipment and raw materials for these processes will be greater than that of traditional agricultural methods. Finally, the protein from soya beans and other similar plants has now, in the middle 1970s, been purified, textured and flavoured to resemble meat. But it is much cheaper to prepare and eat the original beans, with little difference in palatability of the final product. Textured vegetable protein (TVP)is, to my mind, yet another triumph of scientific ingenuity over common sense!

9

Elements and inorganic compounds in diet

So far, in their chemical nature, the foods that we have discussed have all been *organic* compounds, chemicals containing the elements carbon, hydrogen, oxygen and nitrogen. Most common proteins also contain sulphur in cysteine or methionine. Some, such as caseinogen, contain phosphorus and also have calcium attached to them. Phosphorus is also present in nucleoproteins. Iron is attached to other proteins. In this chapter we will consider these and other chemicals or elements that appear in food analyses as *ash*. That is to say, these substances are left behind when the carbon, hydrogen and nitrogen have all been burnt away by excess oxygen.

We need a convenient term for these. No chemical term is entirely suitable, but *inorganic materials* has been chosen. It is not a good name, for although all the elements concerned do appear in inorganic chemistry—i.e. in ores etc. which are mined—they do not always appear in the food or function in the body as inorganic compounds. They should not be called *mineral salts*, because they may not be present in the food as salts. For example the body obtains its sulphur as the amino acids cysteine and methionine. Sulphates cannot be absorbed from the gut and act as purgatives. The term *minerals* is as bad, for it calls up a picture of coal or limestone in one's food!

Apart from sulphur, all the essential materials can be absorbed from the gut (and therefore be present in the food) as inorganic salts. There is no point in giving calcium as the expensive gluconate salt when common chalk is available. Ferric ammonium citrate, a favourite organic iron salt, is far less absorbable than the cheap inorganic ferrous sulphate—indeed, the conditions in the gut probably convert all the iron into the ferrous state. The amounts of the different inorganic materials found in the human body, and in our foods, have an extraordinary range. An adult man may have over 1 kg of calcium in his body, whereas of chromium he has only 5–10 mg and of copper 150 mg. The amounts of some of these materials in the average adult are given in Table 9.1. The amounts of others e.g. cobalt, silicon, tin, molybdenum, selenium and fluorine present in the body are small, but there is evidence that their presence may be required. Cadmium, lead and mercury are three substances, frequently present in our environment, including food, which are quite inessential in any amounts, but which are poisonous to living tissues, and will accumulate in them during life. Thus many adults may contain 20–30 mg of cadmium.

All the substances listed in Table 9.1 and those mentioned above as probably being required by a living body enter into the fluids, cells and

Table 9.1 The amounts of elements other than
carbon, hydrogen, oxygen and nitrogen found
in the human body.

Calcium	1050g
Phosphorus	700g
Potassium	245g
Sulphur	175g
Chlorine	105g
Sodium	105g
Magnesium	35g
Iron	2.8g
Zinc	2.5g
Manganese	210mg
Copper	125mg
Iodine	35mg
Chromium	7.5mg

other structures of the body and may be needed in definite amounts for the proper functioning of these fluids, cells or structures. Thus sulphur is found in cell structures, contractile and other proteins, potassium in cell fluid and sodium in circulating and extra-cellular fluids. It is necessary to the functions of both cells and fluids that the potassium and sodium should stay where they are normally found, and in the normal amounts.

The elements which are found in small amounts (less than 5 g) are probably working as catalysts or in a similar capacity. Except for the special cases picked out in the next section there is, so far, little evidence that we need to concern ourselves with these materials in diets for healthy people. Any substance, listed in Table 9.1 or text, to which we do not refer again is one about which no further significant information is known.

Important trace elements

Cobalt is a constituent part of a vitamin, cobalamin (B_{12}) which will be discussed in the next chapter. No other role is known for cobalt.

Copper is a component of many enzymes, and is required also for mobilisation of iron from its stores as ferritin (of which more later). Children probably need 0.05 mg/kg body weight/day and the adult intake is probably 2 mg/day. Green vegetables, fish and liver are good sources. Milk is poor in copper and the liver of a pregnant mother loses copper to the fetus' liver to tide the new-born infant over the first few months of life. A premature born infant may not receive all of this copper and may thus become deficient. If copper accumulates in the body it is poisonous, especially to the liver and some parts of the brain. This happens if the liver fails to make a special copper transporting protein, caeruloplasmin. Happily, these patients can now be given D-penicillamine, which serves the same function, but the treatment must be continued for life.

Fluorine is essential for the production of hard, caries-resistant enamel in the teeth, but where present in water supplies in more than 3–5 mg/l it causes mottling of the enamel. At over 10 mg/l, calcification of ligaments and tendons may occur, leading to disability. A concentration of 1 mg/l water provides enough to so harden dental enamel as to halve the incidence of dental decay. I find it surprising that this great reduction in a disease state that causes a considerable pain and other problems is not considered by the British population and its rulers to be worth the marginal loss of freedom entailed in ensuring that all our water supplies have at least 1 mg fluorine per litre. Experiments are no longer, in 1977, needed to prove the case. Application of the results is required.

Iodine Of the 25–50 mg of iodine in the body, 8 mg is found in the thyroid gland in the neck, and in areas of the world where the soil and local produce are iodine-deficient, a great swelling of this gland, producing a *goitre*, occurs. This results because the thyroid gland incorporates iodine into its hormone, thyroxine, an essential metabolic regulator substance in the body. If iodine intake is small and not enough thyroxine is being formed, the thyroid gland is stimulated to grow. Probably somewhere between 50 and 300 μg iodine are needed daily in the food to enable an adult to make all the thyroxine he needs. The amount obtained from all land plant and animal foods depends on geological chance—how much iodine the soil happens to contain. In the Mendip hills of Somerset, along the Cotswold and Pennine hills and in the Lake District of England soils are iodine poor, as they are in a wide area around the Great Lakes of N. America, and in the Austrian and Swiss Alps. Common table salt, can have the necessary minute amount of sodium iodine added to it by the manufacturer (such salt is sold in some British grocer's shops), or one can eat small amounts of any sea produce. Thus codfish contains 120 μg/100 g, herring contains 200 μg and salmon 140 μg and shellfish are in the same range. So 150 g, one small herring, contains, at the outside, between one and five days' supply of iodine.

Manganese is a component of some enzymes, but foods such as whole cereal grains or flour, pulses and leafy vegetables ensure such a rich food supply that deficiency has never been observed in man.

Molybdenum may be concerned in iron metabolism and is certainly involved in the metabolic breakdown of nucleoprotein derivatives. Again, human deficiency has never been detected, for in the small amounts needed the diet is always more than adequate.

Zinc is a component of many enzymes essential for normal body function. About 4 mg may be lost daily in the urine and the normal daily diet contains 10–15 mg. Foods rich in zinc are meats, whole cereals and pulses. Fruits and leafy vegetables are poor. Zinc is among the metals bound by the phytic acid present in wheat bran, so some of the whole cereal zinc is not absorbed. In some chronic skin ulcers, healing is accelerated by greatly increasing the oral intake of zinc, as zinc sulphate, but the link between this and the known place of zinc in the bodily economy is not known.

Substances needed in more than trace amounts

Sodium and chlorine

These have been put together because they so frequently occur together as common salt, sodium chloride, in the living body, in the cooking and eating of food, and in the physical world in sea water and rocks. In both physiology and nutrition it is the sodium that matters, for it is sodium that is actively transferred across cell membranes, from the gut, in the kidneys and between tissue fluids and all cells of the body, and it is on various sodium transfer mechanisms that regulatory mechanisms operate. If we look after the sodium, then the chlorine looks after itself! Of course, one has to remember that in the living body it is neither sodium, a fiercely reactive metal, nor chlorine, a reactive and poisonous gas with which we are concerned, but the electrically charged sodium and chloride *ions*, which are quite harmless, as is common salt, the product of combination of sodium and chlorine. When salt dissolves in water, some of its molecules become sodium and chloride ions. This happens in the body with no harm at all to us.

In fact the concentration of salt, the amount of sodium and chloride ions in body fluids is quite critical for normal body function. It is important therefore, to consider the salt intake in the food and salt removal from the body in the urine and sweat. Normally, in temperate climates, so much salt is used in cooking and at the table, and so much is present naturally in our foodstuffs that the supply far exceeds the body's needs, and it is all excreted in the urine. Bacon, cheese, kippers, tinned meats, butter and margarine all contain salt to aid their preservation. Bread, biscuits and breakfast cereals all have salt or bicarbonate added to them. In fact, it is difficult to avoid salt, as you would find if you had to prepare a low salt diet for anyone.

The body needs the salt to maintain the volume and osmotic pressure of tissue fluids and of the blood. Sodium aids carbon dioxide transport in the blood and the conduction of nerve impulses. In Addison's disease (a destruction of the adrenal gland), the kidneys lose their power of retaining sodium in the body, and many of the features of this disease are mimicked by a low salt regime, or by excessive loss of salt through the sweat in a hot climate or hot working conditions. Such a person is listless, mentally impaired, easily fatigued and pants vigorously on taking exercise. Muscular cramps may occur. The state may be seen in coal miners, steel workers, any European moving to a tropical environment, and in babies and the elderly in Great Britain in a hot summer like 1976 when some intercurrent illness affects their dietary salt intake.

In Britain the average intake of 15 g/day is much more than that needed for normal life, but in Burma during the 1939–45 war it was found that nearly 50 g might be lost daily in the sweat. This had to be replaced, by mouth, if the people living and working there were to remain in good health. This has been recognised (though not with such numerical precision) since the days of the Roman Empire. The importance of salt was so well recognised that Roman soldiers were paid partly in salt (salarium) whence comes our modern word 'salary'!

Excess salt accumulates in the body in some kidney diseases and in some diseases of the heart and the liver. Because of its osmotic effect, salt excess invariably leads to water accumulation and *oedema* or dropsy develops. Some people think that mild degrees of salt and water excess leads to the development of a raised blood pressure. Oedema can easily be reduced by restricting sodium intake in the food, and this treatment may also lower a raised blood pressure even in the absence of oedema. Naturally, low salt diets should only be prescribed by a doctor and should only be followed under medical supervision.

Potassium
This is found within the cells of bodily tissues, but not in extracellular fluids. Thus muscle has 0.32% potassium while blood plasma has only 0.01%. When the kidneys re-absorb sodium into the blood they lose a little potassium, but the minimal daily potassium loss may approach zero. A normal full diet contains about 3 g, and this amount is then lost in the urine daily. Most foods have 100–300 mg/100 g, the exceptions being cream, fats, egg white and tripe, white bread and polished rice, which are low in potassium. Only very rarely is it necessary to restrict a patient's intake of potassium, but excessive loss occurs not infrequently and the normal level may be restored by taking potassium rich foods by mouth.

Sulphur
This enters the body as the sulphur-containing amino acids, methionine and cysteine. It is also present in the vitamin, thiamine. The amino acids are required for protein synthesis and connective tissue materials, such as the choudroitin sulphate of cartilage. In a mixed diet there is little shortage of sulphur, as proteins from eggs, meat, milk and cereals all contain over 1% sulphur. Egg and milk proteins have 1.62 and 1.73% respectively, and this is largely as methionine. This amino acid is particularly important in tissue growth and regeneration after illness or injury.

Calcium and phosphorus
These two are considered together because they are both present in bone, in blood they have an important reciprocal relationship, and the high phosphorous content of some foods prevents calcium absorption. Both phosphorus and calcium have, though, many important roles in the body, independent of each other. Thus calcium is concerned with nerve impulse transmission, muscle contraction and blood clotting among its many important roles, while phosphorus is found in the molecules of the nucleic acids that transmit inheritance and build proteins, and it is intimately concerned with energy transfer and storage. In all living tissues phosphorus is present as *phosphate*, one phosphorous atom linked to four oxygen atoms and through them to metal ions such as sodium, potassium or calcium or to organic molecules, such as sugars, and purine or pyrimidine molecules in nucleic acids, for example. At the slightly alkaline state of tissue fluids or blood, calcium phosphate is not very soluble, so the concentration of each

ion sets a limit to the concentration of the other and regulating mechanisms exist that ensure no unwanted deposition of calcium phosphate crystals in the body.

While there may be parts of the world where there is too little phosphorus in the soil or herbage for cattle, human dietary deficiency has rarely been described. All foods contain phosphorus (as phosphate), and dairy foods, fish and meat contain the most, followed by whole grain cereals. In fact, so unimportant is it to be worried about the phosphorus content of food that earlier editions of *The Composition of Foods* left it out of their tables. While the saying, *if we look after the calcium in our diet, the phosphorus will look after itself* may very well be true, the converse is not. Phosphorus is present in the compound phytic acid, which occurs in wheat and rice bran. Phytic acid, if not destroyed, will react with calcium in the intestine and prevent its absorption, so looking too well after the phosphorus in the diet may hinder the calcium uptake from the food.

Calcium enters the body in the food and some is inevitably lost each day in the faeces and in the urine. A balance exists in healthy and adequately fed people between the dietary intake and the losses. If bone growth is occurring in childhood or pregnancy, then the intake has to rise to meet these needs as well as the inevitable losses in urine and faeces. If milk or sweat is being secreted, calcium enters these secretions, and this calcium must be equalled by an increased intake of calcium from the food if the balanced state is to be maintained. The amount of dietary calcium required to achieve balance has been and still is the subject of dispute and research. The DHSS recommended, in 1969, 500 mg for adult men and women, 700 mg for boys and girls during puberty, and 1200 mg for women in the latter 6 months of pregnancy and while producing milk. The latter figure should, perhaps, also be suggested for men who sweat vigorously while working hard in hot environments. But a diet containing only 200 mg in Indian children still allowed the daily accumulation of 77 mg in their bodies, and a Norwegian adult was studied who reduced the calcium intake from 942 mg to 445 mg daily. After 30 weeks he had lost 18.5 g calcium but thereafter remained in balance.

On a diet containing 1000 mg of calcium, 200–300 mg may be absorbed and the rest lost in the faeces. Once in the body this enters a pool, in blood and body fluids, of some 4–7 g. This pool is continuously exchanging calcium with the calcium of bone. There is over 1 kg of calcium in bone as calcium hydroxyapatite (formula $Ca_{10}(PO_4)_6(OH)_2$), and about 700 mg of calcium is daily removed from and added to this material. The urinary loss of calcium is withdrawn from the 4–7 gram pool in the blood, as are any losses in sweat or milk. The pool is maintained constant by two mechanisms. One is the action of hormones which control the rate of calcium deposition into and resorption from bone. The other is the action of a hormone which controls the rate of calcium absorption from the food in the gut. This hormone is liberated by the kidneys when the blood calcium concentration falls. The hormone is made, in two stages by the liver and the kidneys from *cholecalciferol*, recognised for many years as vitamin D, itself to be described in the next chapter. The liver and the kidneys each add a *hydroxyl* (OH) group to the cholecalciferol molecule and the latter organs liberate it when more calcium is required.

The main dietary sources of calcium are milk and cheese. Meats, except tripe, are poor in calcium, fish is moderately good, especially small fish in which the bones are eaten, but cereals, fruit and most vegetables contain but little. It is worthwhile to take the M R C tables, given in *The Composition of Foods* (McCance & Widdowson, 1967), examine the column for calcium per 100 g as purchased and note those foods containing about 100 g or more. These are all breads and biscuits made with flour to which, by government order, calcium is added (as calcium carbonate), dairy produce (except butter and cream), shellfish, herrings, sprats, whitebait, and pilchards, dried figs, almonds and brazil nuts, raw pulses, spring onions, parsley, spinach, watercress and black treacle. Some of the cereal products, the pulses and the dried figs contain phytic acid. It seems then that, for practical purposes, for a constant supply of calcium in the diet we must rely on milk and cheese and the fat fish, not forgetting the oddities like watercress, parsley, black treacle and tripe! In fact, a close correlation has been found between the milk and the calcium intakes in many individual dietary surveys.

It is not surprising to find that the intake of calcium is now deficient in all classes of society. For school children the intake was, at a stroke, reduced by 240 mg/day when the school milk distribution was stopped by government order. This was half to one-third of their daily requirement. In a survey of 120 pregnant women only one reached the recommended calcium intake, and this was because she drank over 1 litre of milk each day. 17 reached 1 g of calcium per day and in many this also was due to a high milk intake. During and for many years after the 1939–45 war, various steps were taken in Britain to encourage pregnant women, nursing mothers and children to drink plenty of milk, the most important being price reduction. Since then, it has been believed that with growing general prosperity these measures are no longer needed. There is a need for further dietary surveys to see whether this belief is well- or ill-founded. If all people could afford to and did drink a pint of milk a day, as the advertising slogan advised, then they would be near to the desired amount.

If we study the imaginary diet first described in Table 5.3, we can see the sources of the dietary calcium (Table 9.2). The total of 1376 mg is largely due to the milk and cheese. Remove these and this day's food contains only 371 mg. Remove the added chalk from the bread and you lose 190 mg of calcium. If you replace the fortified white flour with natural 100% stone ground flour for bread making, the 250 g of bread would contain 60 mg of calcium and enough phytic acid to remove much of the calcium of the milk and cheese. If 50 g of meat is replaced with 50 g of tinned pilchards 3 mg of calcium would be lost and 132 gained. If 25 g of watercress replaced 25 g of cabbage there would be a net gain of 37 mg. One other source of calcium is worth mentioning, and that is hard water. A litre of London water contains 213 mg of calcium. Vegetables boiled in such water will gain little calcium

Table 9.2 The sources of calcium and iron in
a day's food.

		Calcium mg	Iron mg
Bread	250g	230	4.75
Milk	500ml	600	0.35
Bacon	75g	10	0.91
Egg	50g	268	1.27
Meat	125g	6	5.40
Cheese	50g	405	0.29
Butter	50g	8	0.18
Potatoes	100g	9	0.70
Cabbage	100g	75	0.88
Jam	25g	3	0.26
Sugar	50g	2	nil
Total		1376	14.99

from it. But when hard water is boiled in making tea or coffee it loses its calcium. A litre of Burton beer contains about 100 mg of calcium.

More should be said here about the two substances known to precipitate calcium from the food and prevent its absorption. The first is oxalic acid. Oxalates are present in spinach, sorrel and rhubarb. These form small amounts of oxalic acid in the stomach which, if any soluble calcium salt is present, will promptly precipitate as calcium oxalate. The other substance that has already been mentioned several times is phytic acid. In plants this is usually present as calcium magnesium inositol hexaphosphate. In the stomach the highly acid medium splits off the calcium and magnesium, forming their chlorides, but once the food enters the small gut and the acidity is largely neutralised then dicalcium phytate (dicalcium inositol hexaphosphate) is formed, which is even more insoluble than the calcium magnesium phytate. Phytic acid is present in whole cereals, their products and in pulses and other foods as already mentioned. When these form an appreciable part of the diet added calcium must be taken in some form. It has been estimated that 250 g of wholemeal bread prevents absorption of the calcium in 250 ml of milk. It has been suggested that in some circumstances phytic acid digesting enzymes, *phytases*, may develop to reduce the effect of dietary phytates on calcium absorption.

In the 1970s it was noted that there was a negative relationship between hardness of water and disease of the arteries of the heart. Where the water supply was hard, or richer in calcium salts, the incidence of coronary thrombosis and coronary artery disease was lower. As yet there is no explanation for this relationship. It is *not* here being suggested that a raised calcium intake directly protects the coronary arteries from disease processes.

Magnesium
Of the 25 g magnesium in the body, about 5 g is present within the living

cells, where it is mostly found in enzymes, particularly those associated with oxidation of foods and the transfer of energy. Like potassium, magnesium is lost from cells in states of chronic water and salt loss from the tissue fluids and blood, as in some long-standing intestinal disease with diarrhoea. It is also lost excessively in alcoholics. Normally about 300 mg is lost daily in the urine and, since we remain normally in balance, 300 mg is present in a normal diet. Most foods contain a useful amount of magnesium, since it is an essential component in chlorophyll in green plants, no less than in oxidation enzymes in animals. The foods low in magnesium are butter, cream, honey and white sugar. The phytate content of whole cereals etc. will prevent magnesium absorption just as it blocks calcium absorption.

Strontium

Strontium is a metal so like calcium that, though it is sparsely present in soils and foods, it is invariably treated by living bodies *as if it were* calcium, except that there is some evidence that the kidneys, especially of infants, excrete strontium in preference to calcium. All vertebrate bones contain small amounts of strontium, built into the hydroxyapatite crystals of the bone, and they have done so since bone first appeared over 200 million years ago. Since 1945 this has had a new and wholly dangerous significance. Radioactive strontium is a by-product of nuclear weapons and or uranium fission in atomic piles. Some of this inevitably escapes into the environment, enters food chains and ultimately gets deposited in bone. The radiation the strontium gives off there will eventually damage tissues, shorten life and probably cause inheritable defects which may emerge at any time in succeeding generations. From being a perfectly harmless passenger handled largely by living bodies as if it were calcium, strontium has become a sinister by-product of human inventiveness. It enters the body in food, along with our calcium and it may be that, when a region has become heavily contaminated with radioactive strontium, steps will have to be taken to limit the dietary intake of calcium-containing foods produced in that region.

Iron

Iron is part of the haemoglobin in blood, which accounts for two-thirds of the body's iron content. Blood haemoglobin concentration is therefore usually taken as an index of the amount of iron in the body. While the normal amount of haemoglobin in the blood is 14.5 g/100 ml blood, the word 'normal' needs some explaining. For several years now, the incoming medical, dental and science students entering the Physiology department at University College, Cardiff have had their blood haemoglobin measured. For the girls the average is normally between 14 and 14.5 g, but for the boys it is between 15.6 and 15.9 g. In other studies, other average values have been found. For sample populations drawn from both industrial and agricultural areas in South Wales the adult men had an average of 14.5 g and the menstruating women one of 12.5 g/100 ml blood. It has always been thought that the lower figures for women are due to the continual loss of iron in the menstrual flow, that the resultant stimulus to haemoglobin formation is continually active, but that the haemoglobin content of the blood could never reach 14.5 g because of a shortage of iron. Medication with iron and all the other substances known to assist haemoglobin formation may raise the blood haemoglobin somewhat, but seldom to as high as the 'normal' male value. The stimulus to haemoglobin formation seems to 'switch off' at a lower point. Indeed, in some women it may never be possible to raise the haemoglobin above 10 or 11 g/100 ml blood.

Iron is continually lost from the body in urine, sweat, and in shed epithelial cells from skin and gut. Altogether, in men, about 1 mg is lost daily. Women may lose 30 mg in the menstrual flow, so their loss averages over the months at about 2 mg/day. During the 300 (about) days of a human pregnancy, 400 mg iron enters the fetus, 500 enters the placenta and some is inevitably lost in blood lost during labour. A woman's loss through a full-term pregnancy is thus in excess of 3 mg/day in addition to the 1 mg/day of the adult man.

The dietary intake of iron was found in Great Britain in 1971 to average 13.5 mg per person. Table 9.2 shows the iron content of the previously used specimen 1 day's intake of food. This contains the very respectable amount of 15 mg. In fact, although I have chosen average values for the iron content of the sample foods, there is a wide range of iron content. This depends partly on the soil and other factors in food production.

The British (DHSS, 1969) and American (NAS, 1974) estimates of dietary iron requirements differ somewhat, the latter, as is so often the case, being some 20% above the former. Table 9.3 shows the British estimates. The average daily intake in 1971 then appears to be more than enough for all except late adolescent boys and girls, pregnant and nursing women.

Table 9.3 The estimated daily requirement of dietary iron (DHSS, 1969).

Children	0–1 year	6mg	Women	18 years–menopause	12mg
Children	1–3 years	7mg	Women	after the menopause	10mg
Children	3–7 years	8mg			
Children	7–9 years	10mg	Women	4–9 months of	
				pregnancy	15mg
Boys	9–12 years	13mg	Women	Breastfeeding	15mg
and	12–15 years	14mg			
Girls	15–18 years	15mg	Men	Above 18 years	10mg

Why are the dietary requirements so much more than the daily losses? This is because much of the dietary iron is not available for absorption, and because the absorption mechanism is in some way sensitive to the state of the stored iron (ferritin) in the body. If the ferritin stores are full, dietary iron is rejected, and absorption only occurs when the stores are depleted. Oxalates in spinach and, above all, phytic acid in cereals prevent iron absorption by the formation of insoluble iron oxalate or phytate. The iron in meat, in haemoglobin and other similar compounds is only partially absorbed. Thus 15% of the iron in calf liver and 20% of the iron in veal is absorbed, but only 10% of that in fish or haemoglobin. The iron of eggs is poorly absorbed while among vegetables 6% of the iron in soya beans is absorbed. There is some suggestion that the presence of meat raises the iron absorbed from vegetable sources.

Many cereal products, and all British flour, contain added iron. This began as an emergency measure during the 1939–45 war. Prior to that the iron content of the diet was such that about half of all children, 20% of adult men and 60% of women between 26 and 45 years old, all in the South London suburban region of Peckham, were anaemic. Unfortunately, the iron added to flour is finely divided metallic iron, which is now known not to be absorbed by the human intestine. It is therefore useless as a dietary supplement.

When one considers individual items of the specimen day's diet, and their possible replacement, the intake of 15 mg can be varied considerably. 100 g of salad vegetables contain from 1.24 to 4.54 mg iron/100 g and none will be lost to cooking water. 25 g of black treacle instead of jam would provide 2.3 mg instead of 0.26 mg iron. Haricot beans, when cooked, have the same energy content as potatoes, but 2.50 mg iron/100 g, compared with 0.70 mg in potatoes.

The iron content of human milk, like cow's milk, is low and the breast-fed infant relies on the iron store transferred towards the end of pregnancy to see him through the first few months of independent life. It is now customary to add absorbable iron to most proprietary brands of baby milks and cereal feeds. These latter, and other foods are now commonly fed to infants after 3 months and if such foods as green vegetables (other than spinach), minced liver and meat are given, the infant should not become iron deficient.

But as a whole community, we must remember that until the 1940s, Britain was iron-deficient and therefore anaemic. Dietary iron-deficient anaemia has vanished in the wealthier state of Britain in the 1950s, 1960s and the 1970s. One must remember that while anaemia of the iron-deficient type still occurs, it is almost invariably due to excessive blood loss or deficient iron absorption due to a disease in the gut. Only very rarely will we, nowadays, find a person living on a diet that is iron-deficient in Great Britain. In other countries, due to economic or social reasons, dietary iron deficiency is still present and contributes to the anaemia often found there. If such economic stringency were to return to Britain that all the household's meat went to 'working men' and none to the housewife, then, once again she would develop iron-deficient anaemia as did her grandmother in the 1920s and 1930s.

Acid–base equilibrium

The solid end-products of metabolism of a food may be either acidic or alkaline (basic). Thus meat, which is predominantly protein, gives acid end-products; fruits, even those that taste very acid, and vegetables almost all give basic end-products. Proteins contain sulphur and nucleoproteins also contain phosphorus. The sulphur is oxidised to sulphuric acid, while the phosphorus is already present as phosphoric acid, partly neutralised by organic oxidisable materials. These acids are neutralised in the body by basic materials such as sodium and potassium, forming neutral salts (sodium and potassium phosphate and sulphate). These reactions make blood and body fluids slightly more acid. This can only proceed a little way, for life is incompatible with a change of the blood from its normal alkaline state to neutrality (a pH shift from 7.42 to 6.97). The kidneys dispose of the non-gaseous acid substances, which is the cause of the acidic urine seen on a normal diet, rich in animal protein, or when fasting, even overnight. Why fruits, which taste acid, give rise to alkaline end-products, needs some explanation. The acidity of fruit is due to organic oxidisable acids, like citric acid and malic acid. These are present partly as free acid and partly as potassium salts. The free acid and that partly neutralised by potassium are oxidised and the very weakly acid carbon dioxide is blown off in the lungs in the usual way. The potassium combines with some of the carbon dioxide, forming the weakly alkaline potassium bicarbonate. This makes the blood slightly alkaline and is excreted by the kidneys, producing a more strongly alkaline urine.

There is in all this an amusing double paradox. Foods which are neutral or even faintly alkaline (fresh meat or eggs) give rise to an acid urine whereas foods which are definitely acid to litmus produce an alkaline urine. Other acid-producing foods include whole cereals. Milk and all vegetables are alkali-producing, like the 'acid' fruit already mentioned. In any case, in the healthy *it doesn't matter at all whether one eats acid or alkali-producing foods*. The respiratory system and the kidneys are designed to cope with all the alterations in bodily acid/base balance that we can possibly induce by dietary means. As with the excretion of the nitrogenous waste products of protein metabolism, the kidneys cope with any excess of acid that even the high protein diet of the Eskimo or Masai can give them. It is only when the kidneys lose their power to excrete acid due to chronic disease states that one needs to restrict the intake of acid-producing foods. The muddle headed 'food reformers' who tell us to protect the kidneys by avoiding what they believe to be acid-producing, would restrict our intake of fruits such as oranges and lemons which turn the urine alkaline and, moreover, provide us with ascorbic acid.

10
The vitamins

Everywhere in the body we find catalysts acting on the host of chemical reactions that make up the function of living cells. While these are protein substances or enzymes, many require simpler compounds as 'co-factors'. Some of these latter are inorganic substances such as calcium or iron, others are made freely in the body and are used to regulate metabolic processes, others again have to be provided in the food, for they cannot be made in the living body. Thus adrenaline and thyroxine are made in and secreted from the adrenal and thyroid glands and regulate various cellular reactions. For both, the amino acid tyrosine is needed, and thyroxine also contains iodine. Both of these, as we have already seen, must be supplied in the food.

The organic co-factors that we cannot make ourselves are termed the *vitamins*. Sometimes closely related materials, precursors to actual vitamins may be present in the food. They are called *provitamins*.

Vitamins were discovered late in the history of nutrition, for most are present in food in small amounts and their daily requirements are measured in milligrams or micrograms, not in grams. They are irregularly distributed in foods, belonging to no particular class of organic compound. Accurate and painstaking research was needed to identify their existence, to prepare the chemically pure substances, to find their chemical natures and to discover their metabolic functions. They were initially discovered by three converging lines of research: the study of diseases in people living on restricted diets, the discovery of similar diseases in animals, and the feeding of highly purified foodstuffs first to animals and then to people.

As an example we may take the disease beri-beri, in which nerve impulse conduction fails, leading to muscular paralysis and loss of sensation in the skin. The disease was found to be associated with a diet containing a great preponderance of white, polished rice. A Japanese admiral found it could be prevented by providing a more varied diet. Similarly, chickens or pigeons fed on a diet which caused beri-beri in man also developed a disease due to nerve impulse failure. This could be cured by adding to the diet some rice bran, or even a watery extract of rice bran. In Britain it was found that laboratory rats, fed on purified fats, proteins and carbohydrates and sources of inorganic materials, failed to grow and showed signs of muscular paralysis. These signs could be prevented if, to the artificial diet, a small amount of yeast extract, milk or swede juice were added. These three lines of work were brought together in 1912, simultaneously in Britain and Germany, and it was concluded that some essential food factor, not protein, fat, carbohydrate or inorganic material was present in very small amounts in rice bran, yeast, milk and swede juice. This substance was named provisionally *vitamine*, an amine essential to life. The name remains, but the terminal *e* is removed for many of the vitamins are not chemically amines.

It soon became clear that there was not one vitamin but several. One was present in fats and protected the eyes against disease, another was water-soluble, destroyed by heat and protected against paralysis, a third was present in citrus fruits and prevented scurvy. They were given letters of the alphabet, A, B and C respectively. A second fat soluble material was then detected. It prevented rickets and was given the letter D. In the middle 1920s B was found to contain more than one substance, so it was divided into B_1 and B_2. By 1945 there were 10 known materials in the original B vitamin and two more were identified shortly after. Two further fat-soluble vitamins were detected in the 1930s and given the letters E and K.

Once the chemical structures and the functions of the various vitamins were identified, the letter system was replaced by chemical names which indicate the site of action, chemical nature or disease prevented by the vitamin. Vitamin A has become retinol; B_1, which prevented beri-beri is aneurine (preventing neuritis) or thiamine because it contains sulphur; while vitamin C is called ascorbic acid because it prevents scurvy, the Latin name for which is *scorbutes*.

As well as knowing what diseases were prevented by which vitamins, it became essential to know how much of a vitamin any food contained. Before accurate chemical analysis became available, special units of activity were invented and internationally adopted in the 1930s by the League of Nations. *International Units* are still used to express the contents of some vitamins in foods, but we are increasingly using actual weights—milligrams or micrograms per 100 gram portion of the food being considered. This is the system that will be used in this book. We may find that several related chemicals have the same vitamin activity, or are a third or half as active as the vitamin itself. In these cases the food composition tables speak of, for example, retinol (vitamin A) equivalent.

It is very fortunate that, for practical purposes, we do not have to pay attention to all the vitamins hitherto discovered. Those found first are the ones still most likely to be absent from a diet and if the intake of these is satisfactory, it is most unlikely that we will go short of those more recently discovered. Exceptions exist to this, as to any other rule and these will be mentioned in the following descriptions. In these, the fat-soluble vitamins are taken first, then ascorbic acid and finally the compounds originally included in vitamin B.

Retinol

This substance was originally known as vitamin A. Its ability to protect epithelia from infection endowed it with the name *anti-infective vitamin* and it was for a while called *axerophthol* (because it prevented dryness of the eyes).

In foods it is present either as the preformed vitamin or as a provitamin, many of which are found in vegetable foods. These provitamins are highly coloured and belong to the carotene group of vegetable dyes. *Carotene* takes its name from carrots, for it is the orange coloured material in these vegetables. It also occurs with chlorophyll in all green vegetables, though the chlorophyll masks the colour of carotene. Yellow-coloured fruits, such as peaches, apricots and oranges, and vegetables such as some sweet potatoes and pumpkins also owe their colour to carotene. Cryptoxanthine, the red colouring matter of Cape gooseberries and paprika also acts as a provitamin.

The provitamins are changed to retinol during absorption through the intestinal wall, about a third to half the provitamin molecule becoming retinol. The food tables quote either retinol content, or provitamin (carotene) content and the latter must (for safety) be divided by 3 to obtain the equivalent retinol figure.

Absence of retinol or its provitamin from the diet over a period produces changes in the retina of the eyes, epithelial tissues, and in bone.

The retina is the light-sensitive cellular layer at the back of the eyes. It contains cells (rods) that are sensitive to dim light and this sensitivity is due to the substance *rhodopsin* in the rods. Rhodopsin (also called visual purple) is a compound of retinol and protein. Faint light splits the compound and initiates a series of changes that produce nerve impulses. Bright light completely destroys rhodopsin, the retinol being carried away in the blood. Rhodopsin is re-formed in the dark, but *only when* there is sufficient retinol in the blood. Retinol shortage, then, interferes with one's ability to see in the dark and this power is one of the most delicate ways of testing for retinol deficiency (though there are other forms of night blindness not due to this lack).

Epithelium is the name given to the cellular tissue lining the mouth, nose, trachea and bronchi, the digestive and genito-urinary tracts, the inside of eyelids and over the exposed part of the eyeballs, and to the glandular outgrowths of these various tracts and tubes. All epithelia depend upon a supply of retinol if they are to remain in good health and repel bacterial invasions. The epithelial coating of eyelids and eyes, the conjunctiva, together with that of the tear gland are particularly sensitive to retinol shortage, which produces dry, sore eyes, which readily develop bacterial conjunctivitis, Xerophthalmia. Much of the blindness seen in children in poor countries is due to retinol deficiency, and such people also suffer from a low resistance to infection in respiratory and urogenital systems.

Bone, as we grow, is continually being re-shaped, growing in one site and being resorbed in another site. Retinol appears essential for proper bone resorption, especially around the opening in the skull through which the cranial nerves pass. A late sign of retinol deficiency is pinching and degeneration of these nerves. Bone-forming cells (osteoblasts) are present in profusion, but there is a scarcity of bone-absorbing cells (osteoclasts).

The nature of retinol

For those who like to know chemical structural formulae, that of retinol is given here.

```
H₃C        CH₃
   \     /        H   CH₃  H   CH₃  H
     C              |    \   |    \   |
   /     \         C     C    C     C    C – OH
H₂C        C===C    C    C    C    \
 |          ||   |    |    |    |    H
H₂C         C    H    H    H    H
   \      / \
    CH₂       CH₃
```

Since it is so largely composed of carbon and hydrogen, as are fatty substances, it is to be expected that it is soluble in fat and not in water. The one OH group at the end of the chain of carbon atoms puts retinol in the class of alcohols and enables it to combine with fatty acids and other substances.

It is a pale yellow oil, very easily oxidised when exposed to air and heat or ultraviolet light. Such oxidation destroys its biological activity. Ordinary cooking processes, however, do not harm retinol or the carotenes from which it can be formed. Cooking of, for example, carrots enhances their digestibility and so makes more of the carotene available for absorption.

The amounts recommended by the DHSS in 1969 range from 300 μg/day for children between 1 and 7 years old, to 750 μg/day for adult men and women. During lactation 1200 μg daily are recommended. Needless to say, the American recommendations are some 25–30% higher than these! Individuals' needs will vary with the efficiency of absorption.

Retinol itself is present in fish and mammalian livers, the flesh of fatty fish, in milk and eggs. Carotenes etc. are, as already mentioned, widely distributed in small amounts in green and yellow vegetables and fruits. Table 10.1 gives the retinol (or carotene equivalent) content of the specimen day's food intake. Almost all of this derives from milk and its products, and it must be recommended that these are average values only. The retinol content of milk, cheese and butter can fall to two-thirds of these values in winter, or when the cows are on a retinol or carotene low diet. But this day's retinol intake is above the recommended level for an adult, and substitution of the butter by fortified margarine would almost guarantee an adequate intake. Occasional meals of calf or lamb liver, which contain 1200 to 13 500 μg retinol/100 g would give a substantial reserve.

Table 10.2 gives the retinol and the cholecalciferol contents of some of the major foods. From this list it should be clear that it is easy to devise a diet adequate for retinol, and that there are materials from which highly concentrated retinol preparations can readily be made. The human body can store considerable amounts of retinol (presumably in the liver), so an occasional meal of a food containing a large amount can redress several days of less than the recommended intake. In regions where the diet is deficient in the natural foods in this list, small amounts of fish liver oils, or liver from mammals can be used to make up the average daily requirement.

Acute poisoning may be induced by eating polar bear liver, but a more

Table 10.1 The retinol and cholecalciferol contents of a day's food.

		Retinol μg	Cholecalciferol μg
White bread	250g	nil	nil
Milk	500ml	225	0.1
Bacon	75g	trace	trace
Egg	50g	160	0.7
Meat	125g	trace	trace
Cheese	50g	220	0.2
Butter	50g	475	1.0
Potatoes	100g	trace	nil
Cabbage	100g	100	nil
Jam	25g	nil	nil
Sugar	50g	nil	nil
Totals		1180	2.0
Margarine	50g	450	3.8
Calf or lamb liver	125g	1500–17 000	0.6–1.4

Table 10.2 The retinol and cholecalciferol content of foods (μg per 100g).

	Retinol	Cholecalciferol
Halibut liver oil	600 000–10 800 000	500–10 000
Cod liver oil	12 000–120 000	200–750
Polar bear liver oil	600 000	
Fresh herring	25–50	5–45
Tinned salmon and sardine	25–90	5–45
Milk	20–70	0.1
Cheese	360–520	0.3
Butter	720–1200	0.3–2.5
Fortified margarine	900	0.8
Eggs	300–340	1.3–1.5
Lamb liver	3000–30 000	0.5
Ox liver	3000–12 000	1.1
Carrots	600–1500	nil
Green leafy vegetables	?–1200	nil
Red or yellow yams	380–770	nil
White yams	50	nil
Apricots	70–280	nil
Bananas	10–30	nil

common chronic poisoning occurs when parents misguidedly dose their children with halibut liver oil as if it were cod liver oil. Daily doses of 30 000–150 000 (100–500 × requirement) are needed to produce harm. Recovery is rapid following withdrawal of the doses.

Cholecalciferol

The second fat-soluble vitamin, originally called vitamin D, again has two provitamins, each of which can be converted into the active vitamin. The provitamins are sterol compounds, 7-dehydrocholesterol and ergosterol. The former is present in animal fats, including the oily secretions of sebaceous glands and the preening glands of birds. The latter is found in ergot, yeast and other fungi. The provitamins are converted into the active material by ultraviolet light. Therefore one could say that cholecalciferol is not a vitamin at all, since we do not need to take it by mouth. However, the sum doesn't always provide ultraviolet light, particularly in the winter in Britain or when our industrial activities add so much dust, smoke and water vapour to the air that the ultraviolet light cannot reach our skins. It is therefore important to remember that cholecalciferol present in food can replace that which cannot be formed in the skin in the absence of sunlight. Once it is absorbed from skin or gut, cholecalciferol undergoes two further changes before it becomes active. In the liver an OH group is added at the end of the side chain, and in the kidneys, only when the blood level of calcium falls, a second OH group is added at the other end of the molecule. See Fig 10.1 for the structural formulae of these compounds. This compound, 1,25-dehydroxycholecalciferol (1,25 DCC) then travels in the blood to the intestinal lining, where it potentiates the absorption of calcium from the food, provided calcium is available in the digestion mixture. No amount of 1,25 DCC, or of sunlight, will be any use if the dietary calcium is deficient or combined as oxalate or phytate. 1,25 DCC also has a direct action on the kidneys, promoting the resorption of phosphate from the urine. Thus both the calcium and the phosphate concentration of blood are raised, a condition that favours the precipitation of calcium phosphate or hydroxyapatite, the crystalline component of bone.

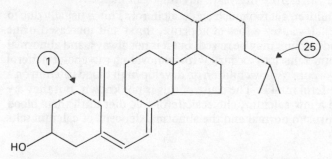

Fig. 10.1 The structural formula of cholecalciferol. The arrows indicate the positions where OH groups are added in the liver (C25) and the kidneys (C1).

Due to the existence of two sources of cholecalciferol, it has not been possible to determine accurately our daily requirement. Most authorities settle for a daily dietary intake of 10 μg, though none would have been needed in the summer months of 1975 and 1976 in Britain. Children living in the tropics whatever their ethnic origin, need none in their food, but children with dark skins living in a temperate climate need their 10 μg each day in their food. The consequence of deficiency is rickets. The bones are poorly calcified and soft, so that limb bones bend under the body weight. The regions where active calcification *should* be occurring become swollen. In severe cases the blood calcium itself falls and abnormalities develop in nerve impulse conduction (tetany). A comparable disease, *osteomalacia* (literally 'softened bones'), is seen in adults. It should be stressed that rickets is a calcium deficiency disease, for it was produced in the 1940s in Eire by the widespread use of wholemeal flower, in which phytic acid prevented calcium absorption. But rickets may be caused by calcium shortage, cholecalciferol shortage or absence of sunlight. All three conditions will be accentuated by poverty in an urban environment in a temperate climate. The diet will be low in both calcium and cholecalciferol, industrial haze and climatic conditions will reduce sunlight. If one adds to these the presence of a dark skin and dietary restrictions and habits (wholemeal flour for chapatti making, for example), it is not surprising that rickets is still with us in Great Britain. The specimen day's diet in Table 10.1, contains only 2.0 μg of cholecalciferol, so it is grossly deficient. This could be raised to 4.75 μg by substituting fortified margarine for the butter, but to an average of 10 μg/day only by a plentiful consumption of the fat fish or of fish liver oils. No other foods have more than a small amount of cholecalciferol. Unfortunately the Peruvian anchovy, the herring and now the mackerel and salmon are being fished so vigorously that they may disappear as completely as the Californian sardine. Some of this fish is converted to meal for animal feed and much of its cholecalciferol content is lost to human consumption. The only certain way to maintain dietary cholecalciferol intake is to incorporate cod or halibut liver oil in white sauces used in preparing fish dishes (such as cod au gratin). Otherwise we have to rely on climatic vagaries which means, in Britain, that over the years anything can happen!

Occasionally children get too much cholecalciferol. This is usually due to parental mistakes. It causes a loss of appetite, thirst and increased urine output. The blood calcium may be raised, but it is not always, and abnormal deposits of calcium salts may occur. With removal of the cholecalciferol source, recovery occurs. A few children do develop high blood calcium on a normal cholecalciferol intake. The cause of this is not known, but they are best treated with a low calcium, cholecalciferol-free diet until their blood calcium level returns to normal and the abnormal deposits of calcium salts have vanished.

The tocopherols

These were discovered in 1923 and labelled vitamin E. They are fat-soluble materials found principally in seed oils, wheat germ oil having the most. Deficiency in rats causes sterility in males and abortion in females. Fatty degeneration and fibrosis also develop in muscles, a condition like human muscular dystrophy.

Since other reasonable sources of tocopherols include dairy produce, eggs and green vegetables, it is not likely that a person with a diet adequate for retinol and other major vitamins will ever suffer tocopherol shortage, so they can be ignored for practical purposes.

Naphthoquinones

These were discovered in 1934 in Denmark and called vitamin K for they were needed for clotting of blood (hence 'koagulations vitamin'). The active compounds are present in some of the clovers, but are readily formed in the human intestine by bacteria normally living there. In health we obtain all the naphthoquinone we need from this source. Naphthoquinone deficiency may occur early in the infancy before the normal intestinal bacteria become established. Milk contains but little pre-formed material. In adults, deficiency may be due to poor absorption from the intestine, or the liver, if severely diseased, may fail to use the absorbed naphthoquinone in making various clotting factors, for naphthoquinones are required in producing 4 of the 10 essential materials for blood clotting. Some similar materials, also produced by clovers, can antagonise the actions of this vitamin, and so reduce the clotting tendency of blood. One of these, *warfarin*, is regularly used in medical treatment and also as a rat poison.

Absorption of fat-soluble vitamins

It should be mentioned here that absorption from the gut of all four of the fat-soluble vitamins is determined by the same factors that determine fat absorption. The bile salts aid fat absorption which, indeed, is grossly defective in their absence, as in biliary tract obstruction. Malabsorption syndrome, coeliac disease and sprue are all associated with defective fat absorption. Fat-soluble vitamin deficiencies may be part of the consequences of these disease states. Finally, some people take 'liquid paraffin' ('mineral oil' in the USA) as a laxative. This completely non-digestible material will dissolve the fat-soluble vitamins and so prevent their absorption from the intestine.

Ascorbic acid

As early as 1601 it was known that oranges and lemons or fresh green vegetables could protect a person against scurvy, a disease that broke out after several weeks or months on a diet devoid of fresh or growing vegetable foods. The disease is characterised by bleeding into the gums which become painful, swollen and infected, bleeding under the skin and into joints which also become swollen and intensely painful. In 1747, a naval surgeon, James Lind compared the curative effects of oranges compared with cider, hydrochloric acid, vinegar, sea water, and 'an electuary . . . made of garlic, mustard seed, *rad. raphan.*, balsam of Peru, and gum myrrh'. Only those who had oranges recovered from the scurvy, which they did within a week.

85°C also inactivates the oxidising enzymes that themselves destroy ascorbic acid. So a short period of cooking, following a rapid rise in temperature may preserve much of the ascorbic acid of the fresh vegetables. Ascorbic acid is dissolved out into the cooking water, so as little as possible should be used, and the vegetables cooked, as far as is convenient, in the steam above the boiling water. The water, ideally, should be brought to the boil and the freshly shredded vegetables added to it at such a rate that it doesn't cease boiling. A close-fitting lid should then cover the pan. For $\frac{1}{2}$ lb (just over 200 g and about 2 medium servings) of chopped cabbage, 2–3 minutes of boiling is sufficient, and preferable, in the author's opinion, to a longer cooking period. A little soda or sodium bicarbonate is often added in cooking of green vegetables to enhance their colour. This may increase the rate of oxidative loss of ascorbic acid.

The keeping of vegetables hot for some time after cooking is very destructive of ascorbic acid. In 15 minutes a quarter of the original amount is lost, and after 90 minutes three quarters. In institutional catering the staff like to get through the cookery as early as possible and keep the cooked foods hot for servings over 1–2 hours. Vegetables served in a restaurant or canteen may have only a third of the ascorbic acid with which they started from the kitchen.

Canning and bottling

Originally much loss was thought to be inevitable, but actual experimentation has shown that canned fruit or vegetables, even after prolonged storage, may actually contain more ascorbic acid than those bought on the open market and cooked at home. The reasons are: (a) none but the best quality material is preserved; (b) the time between picking, and preserving is shorter as it does not include marketing (wholesale and retail), and taking home and cooking, (c) the oxidising enzymes are rapidly destroyed by the 'blanching' process when done on a large scale, and (d) the food is packed and preserved out of contact with oxygen. In these respects, the household bottling process may not be as successful as the industrialised methods. Very similar arguments will apply to the large-scale deep-freezing of vegetables and fruit.

Dehydration

Vegetables and fruits have for centuries been dried as a method of preservation. But slow drying in air provides the best environment for the destruction of ascorbic acid. If the enzymes can be rapidly destroyed and the material dried with little exposure to air, 60–80% of the ascorbic acid can be preserved.

Ascorbic acid content of foods

Among fresh fruit and vegetables, ascorbic acid is very widely distributed, many containing between 20 and 50 mg/100 g. It is simplest to single out the conspicuously high and low values, rather than include a long and indigestible table of all these foods (which would inevitably leave out some favourite foods of every reader!). At the low end, less than 20 mg/100 g, come apples, pears, plums and bananas among fruit, lettuce, cucumber and tomatoes in the salad vegetables, and french beans among green vegetables. Root vegetables, leeks and onions are also low. Among the very high contents, over 50 mg/100 g, come blackcurrants, strawberries and oranges. Cabbages, brussel sprouts, cauliflower and broccoli along with turnip leaves, mustard and bean sprouts are the best of the green vegetables. Potatoes deserve a special mention, because so many people eat a lot of them. Early and freshly dug maincrop potatoes contain 30 mg/100 g. By Christmas the content may be 20 mg, and by spring down to 10 mg/100 g. In all cases, cooking the green vegetables may reduce the ascorbic acid content to a third of the fresh value, but cooking potatoes leaves them with 50–80% of their original content.

Grains and pulses are ascorbic acid free, but once they germinate and sprout the growth is rich in the vitamins. Milk contains 1–2 mg/100 ml, while the livers of various animals contain 20–30 mg. It is upon seal liver that the Eskimo depends for his ascorbic acid, as already mentioned.

Despite this widespread distribution of ascorbic acid among many, readily available foods, it is still possible, even in hospitals, for the actual consumption to fall to below 15 mg/day. Such institutions may prepare the food in ways that destroy the ascorbic acid, or present them in an unpalatable form. Even at home, it is too easy for the single person to develop lazy and stereotyped cooking or eating habits and run short of ascorbic acid. So long as the cabbage vegetables are properly cooked, or one eats an orange each day, scurvy can be as easily prevented as it may be caused by bad habits! The specimen day's diet contains 5–10 mg in the milk, 20 mg from the cabbage after cooking and 5–20 mg from the potatoes, so that was all right! If rice had been substituted for potatoes and root vegetables for the cabbage, then it would have been deficient.

This description of ascorbic acid cannot be completed without some mention of the supposed effects of large doses of the vitamin. While several separate, well-controlled, sets of observations have shown that a well-fed person uses about 45 mg daily, and that he can remain healthy on as little as 10 mg, the studies that claim that 1–2 g daily promotes optimal health, and prevents the development of the common cold have not been confirmed, and the claims rested upon very tenuous foundations. It is, moreover, possible that such large doses may actually be harmful, since they may affect bone metabolism and increase urinary oxalate excretion, with the danger of forming renal stones. Nutritional notions that are not backed by sound reasoning and experimental evidence should be ignored.

Thiamine

This substance is the original water soluble, heat labile vitamin B, also known as aneurine. It prevents the symptoms and signs of beriberi and of similar diseases in animals. Its structural formula is shown below.

$$
\begin{array}{ccc}
 & & \mathrm{CH_3} \\
 & & | \\
\mathrm{N=CNH_2HCl} & & \mathrm{C=C.CH_2.CH_2OH} \\
| \quad | & \qquad\qquad\qquad \diagup & \\
\mathrm{H_3C-C \quad C} \longrightarrow \mathrm{CH_2-N} & | \\
|| \quad || & \diagup \quad \diagdown\diagdown & | \\
\mathrm{N-CH} & \mathrm{Cl} \quad \mathrm{C-S} \\
 & & | \\
 & & \mathrm{H}
\end{array}
$$

The left-hand ring of nitrogen and carbon atoms is one that turns up in many compounds in living tissues, including the nucleic acids, the carriers of genetic information. The right-hand ring, containing carbon, nitrogen and sulphur atoms is but rarely found in living organisms, apart, that is, from thiamine. The substance is an essential co-factor for one of the key enzymes in carbohydrate metabolism. It allows pyruvic acid, the product of non-oxidative breakdown of glucose, to enter the oxidation system, in which 90% of the energy of glucose is released.

Whenever a person eats a thiamine deficient diet he will develop beri-beri. Since in no diet is the vitamin totally absent, the onset of the disease is usually insidious. It starts with excessive fatigue, sensations of heaviness and stiffness in leg muscles, inability to walk far, and abnormal breathlessness on exercise. Sufferers may also complain of mental and mood changes, and later of sensory loss and abnormal sensations from the skin. When examined they may be anaemic, and the heart rate is abnormally fast on exercise. An excess of tissue fluid is seen in the legs—a sign of weakness of the heart muscle.

Since thiamine is so closely concerned in carbohydrate oxidation it is not surprising that thiamine deficiency produces problems mainly related to the one tissue of the body, the nervous system, that uses a carbohydrate oxidation almost exclusively as its source of energy, and that pyruvic acid should appear in the blood in sufferers from beri-beri or in thiamine-deficient animals. Thiamine requirements are also found to be related roughly to total energy turnover and to carbohydrate intake in the diet. In fact, a thiamine:energy ratio was accepted by a joint FAO/WHO committee in 1967. This ruled that for every MJ of energy in the food intake, there should be an intake of 96 μg thiamine, though the critical lower level of sufficiency might be around 60 μg thiamine per MJ of food energy. At this level 480 μg would cover basal energy requirements and 960 μg (0.96 mg) would be just enough for a very energetic person. If one accepts the internationally accepted ratio, this amount is the daily required intake for the normal sedentary person with a daily energy turnover of 10 MJ. The amounts needed for all ages and types of person can be calculated similarly from the accepted thiamine:energy ratio.

While almost all foods contain *some* thiamine, the important sources are plant seeds, yeast, pig meat and offals, though most of us depend almost entirely on cereal foods for our thiamine. In these the processes of milling become very important, for the thiamine is not distributed uniformly throughout the grain. Polished rice and 70% extraction wheat flour are deficient in thiamine as has already been described (Chapter 6, and Table 6.5). Wholemeal bread contains about three times as much thiamine as white bread made from unfortified flour. The thiamine added by the 1956 government order to 70% extraction flour restores most of that lost in the milling process. In the cooking of rice, since thiamine is both soluble and heat-labile, considerable quantities of thiamine are lost, of that which par-boiling before milling had preserved in the white-grain rice. I have found that, with care, by cooking brown rice in three times its own volume of water in a covered pan, the rice is cooked just before it has absorbed all the water and starts sticking to the pan and burning. By this means, I expect to retain a considerable part of the thiamine content. Brown rice has a better flavour than does white rice, anyway, just as wholemeal bread is, to me, preferable to white!

While most meats contain 0.03–0.15 mg thiamine/100 g, bacon and pork contain 0.40–1.0 mg, and offals about 0.30 mg/100 g. Raw ox heart may, however, contain up to 0.6 mg/100 g. Cod roe, for some unexplained reason, contains 1.5 mg, while hens' eggs only 0.1 mg/100 g. Raw haricot beans, peas and lentils contain 0.45, 0.50 and 0.32 mg/100 g, and are outstanding among vegetables for thiamine.

In summary, while it is not easy to go altogether without thiamine, our supply of the vitamin depends on wholemeal or fortified flour, milk, beans etc. and the pig. The specimen day's diet (see Table 10.3) contains enough thiamine, for its 10.36 MJ of energy is covered by 1.19 mg thiamine, whereas 1.0 mg is needed for the accepted ratio.

Nicotinic acid

This substance was known to organic chemists in the nineteenth century,

Table 10.3 Vitamins in a single day's food.

| | | Thiamine | Nicotinic acid | Riboflavine | Folic acid | Cobalamin | Ascorbic acid |
		mg	mg	mg	μg	μg	mg
White bread	250g	0.45	4.3	nil	25	nil	nil
Milk	500ml	0.20	0.4	0.75	1.5	1.5	0–5
Bacon	75g	0.30	1.2	0.12	nil	nil	nil
Egg	50g	0.05	trace	0.18	4.0	0.35	nil
Meat	125g	0.06	6.3	0.28	12.5	2.5	nil
Cheese	50g	0.02	0.6	0.25	nil	1.0	nil
Butter	50g	trace	trace	trace	nil	nil	nil
Potatoes	100g	0.08	0.8	0.03	6.0	nil	5–15
Cabbage	100g	0.03	0.2	0.15	20	nil	10–60
Jam	25g	nil	nil	nil	nil	nil	nil
Sugar	50g	nil	nil	nil	nil	nil	nil
Totals		1.19	13.8	1.76	69.0	5.35	15–70

extracted from yeast and rice bran in the search for thiamine in 1913, but only finally identified as a vitamin in 1933. That a protein-free extract of meat or yeast prevented the human disease of pellagra was known by the middle 1920s, but in some way pellagra seemed to be *caused* by eating maize meal. Finally, by 1933, it was clear that the pellagra-preventing factor of meat or yeast was nicotinic acid or the closely related nicotinamide, that the vitamin could be made in the human body from the amino acid tryptophan (60 mg tryptophan producing 1 mg nicotinic acid), and we now know that the association of pellagra with maize is due to the absence of tryptophan in the maize protein, zein, and to its nicotinic acid being unabsorbable unless (as in Mexican tortilla making) the maize is treated with lime.

The structural formulae of nicotinic acid and of nicotinamide, the form in which it is found in the body are as follows:

$$
\begin{array}{cc}
\text{Nicotinic acid} & \text{Nicotinamide}
\end{array}
$$

Nicotinamide is a component of enzymes associated in all living beings with oxidative metabolism. Pellagra consists of inflammation in the skin and digestive tract (dermatitis and diarrhoea) and changes in the nervous system similar to beri-beri, though in pellagra these have been associated more with a generalised dementia (giving the 3Ds). The earliest indications of the disease are redness of the skin in regions exposed to sunlight and mental dullness. The disease is still common in many regions where maize is the main source of energy in the food.

As with thiamine, it has been found useful to relate nicotinic acid or nicotinamide requirement to the energy needs of people, and the recommended ratio is 1.6 mg/MJ. Thus the normal sedentary adult needs about 16 mg/day and the diet shown in Table 10.3 is about 2.5 mg short of the required amount. This diet, however, contains over 11 g of tryptophan and so can provide the 150 mg needed to make up the nicotinamide deficiency with plenty to spare.

The vitamin itself comes from the fortified flour used to make the white bread and the meat, with smaller contributions from the bacon, potatoes, milk and cheese. The bulk of the tryptophan comes from milk and cheese with sizeable contributions from the meat and the bread. In general, the best sources of this vitamin are wholewheat flour (which contains 4–5.5 mg/100 g, as compared with the 1.0 mg of 70% extraction flour, which is then fortified to 1.5 mg/100 g), meats at 3–6 mg/100 g, and offals at 7–17 mg. Milk, cheese and eggs are poor sources of the preformed vitamin, but their very high tryptophan content makes them valuable sources of nicotinic acid. Lightly milled rice contains 2.0–4.5 mg, pulses 1.5–3 mg and groundnuts 16 mg/100 g. Sage and tapioca (cassava) contain no nicotinic acid. Diets containing wholewheat or unpolished rice contain sufficient nicotinic acid, but if maize, sago or cassava are the chief energy sources, it is the tryptophan content of the protein that provides the nicotinic acid. This must come from meat, fish, dairy products or eggs.

Riboflavin

This vitamin was identified at about the same time as nicotinic acid, but as a growth promoting substance, not as the essential material needed to prevent a specific disease. Like nicotinamide, riboflavin is a component of an enzyme associated with oxidative metabolism.

The structural formula of riboflavine is shown below:

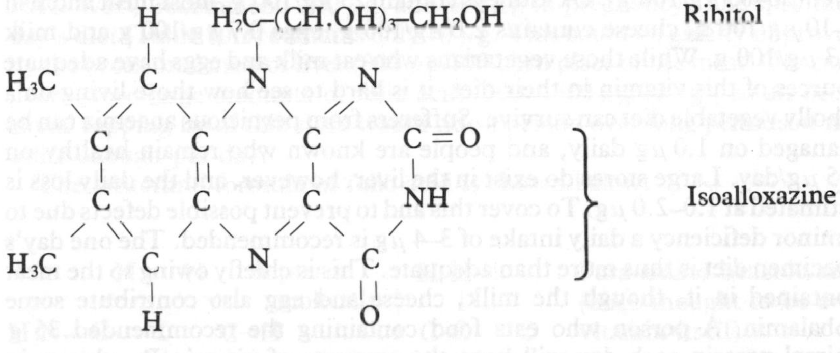

$$H \quad H_2C-(CH.OH)_3-CH_2OH \qquad \text{Ribitol}$$

Isoalloxazine

It is curious that despite the key role of this enzyme in metabolism, no deficiency disease comparable to beri-beri or pellagra develops in riboflavin deficiency. An inflammatory lesion develops at the angles of the mouth, and an appearance like that of chapped lips. Nasolabial seborrhoea also is associated with riboflavin deficiency. This is enlarged and blocked sebaceous glands on the nose, cheeks and forehead. In severe cases, capillary blood vessels invade the corneas of the eyes, with soreness and lacrimation.

The recommended riboflavin intake is 0.13 mg/MJ energy, so the specimen day's diet, containing 1.76 mg, has an excess over the 1.35 mg needed for its energy content of 10.36 MJ. The best sources of riboflavin are liver and kidneys with 2.0–3.0 mg/100 g, cheese and eggs with 0.3–0.5 mg/100 g. Whole grains of wheat and barley contain 0.12–0.25 mg/100 g and meats 0.10–0.30/100 g. Milk contains 0.15 mg/100 g and green vegetables 0.05–0.30 mg/100 g. It is seldom, in fact, that frank deficiency occurs, though there may be many people in the world who approach deficiency through a diet containing little animal, whole grain or green vegetable foods.

11

Some theoretical considerations of scientific nutrition

A problem that worries the scientific dietitian is that nutrition, as applied to human dietetics is no exact science like, for example, physics or chemistry. The practising dietitian has to realise that there are no rigid laws, the application of which results in perfect solutions. For example, oedema (dropsy) due to weakness of the heart muscle is usually treated with a low salt diet, one with plenty of fruit and vegetables and no added salt. But this treatment may not work because of an idiosyncrasy in a particular patient. The following account was related by the late Dr George Graham of St Bartholomew's Hospital in London. 'Polly, an 8-year-old girl, had dropsy due to heart failure. She had vomited all the carefully prepared food given her for several days. In despair the physician said she could eat whatever she liked. Polly chose, and was given, fried sausages. She was not sick, and from that day began a rapid recovery from her dropsy.' At that time, fried pork sausages had over 2% common salt and would have been excluded from any low salt diet. Such an exception to rule will be met from time to time in the practice of dietetics and one should consider some of the reasons for accepting with caution all that has been given in earlier chapters. One should also remember that, even in such striking exceptions as in the story about Polly, a rational and scientific reason for the event awaits discovery.

Dietetics is not, and can never be, an exact science. It has no 'laws' other than the general physico-chemical ones based on conservation of mass and energy. These *are* true for the human body, however much some unorthodox dietitians or overweight people may wish them to be untrue—if a body oxidises more material than it receives in its food and drink it will lose weight. If it requires less energy than is contained in its food, it will gain weight as some of the excess is stored in the fat depots. These two statements we can take as certain. To this extent the living body does behave as a machine, but as a machine with many individual vagaries. No two models are exactly alike, but all differ in many small details, just as, even in the best regulated of production lines, no two cars are precisely the same. We should now study the limitations of the science of nutrition.

Weighing the human body

This cannot be done with the accuracy that a chemist can weigh food. The body's weight changes from moment to moment; even when sitting quietly in a chair the fluctuations may be 14 g, which for a 70 kg man is one part in 5000. When weighed at the same time every day, the day-to-day variations, for a man, may exceed 1.0 kg, perhaps being as much as one part in 50. Yet frequently one sees measurements of, for example, energy output, calculated to four significant figures, one part in 1000. The daily heat output of a person may be given as 8.453 MJ. If the energy equivalent of 100 g pure fat is 3.5 MJ one can see how even a 0.1% error in weighing a person (70 g) might cause a large error in heat output estimates solely from food input. The heat output figure should be given to the same degree of accuracy, usually 1%, of a reliable laboratory balance suitable for weighing people. The figure of 8.453 then becomes somewhere between 8.53 and 8.37. Luckily the daily fluctuations of body weight are usually due to changes in water content, and not fat, so what concerns us is the reliability of immediately repeated weighings of the same person, the figure given above of ± 1.0%.

Food analysis tables

These tables, upon which so much dietetic work relies, cannot be taken as entirely accurate. In the first place, different samples of the same food may differ in their composition. The tables usually give only average values, and it is certain that the bread eaten by the participants of a dietary survey is not the same piece that was analysed by the compilers of the tables. Even bread from the same baker may vary in protein from 7 to 10%.

The figures are much less trustworthy when we come to the vitamins and inorganic materials. The outer leaves of a cabbage have more calcium (and probably iron) than the inner ones, they contain more carotene, but the ascorbic acid is more uniformly distributed. The tables will bluntly say 'cabbage:calcium, 75 mg; iron, 0.9 mg; carotene, 0.3 mg; ascorbic acid, 60 mg per 100 g', and we assume that the cabbage we give someone has just these amounts. Fuller tables do differentiate between 'loose leaf' cabbage—kale, spring cabbage or sprout tops—and headed cabbage (savoy, etc.), giving a carotene content of 5.0 mg for the former and 0.3 mg for the latter.

The ideal would be for all tables to show average values and the range of individual values around this average. Even then it will remain unclear whether a diet could yield, for example, 30 or 60 mg ascorbic acid, or 0.3 or 5.0 mg carotene. Only by determining each constituent of a diet or of aliquot parts of the food eaten could you be sure of what the recipient *puts into his mouth*. Even then it is not possible to know what is absorbed from his gut.

Nutritional requirements

Here I must recapitulate many comments that were made in several earlier chapters concerning the recommended daily intakes of different constituents of foods. The points made in the last section prevent our accepting uncritically any estimates for the amounts of the component foods in any diet, even if drawn up by the foremost of nutritional experts. Many estimates of nutritional needs have been put forward from time to time and accepted as truth by uncritical dietitians. Thus at the beginning of the twentieth century it was believed that the daily need of the average person was for 100 g protein, 100 g fat and 400 g carbohydrate. This replaced an earlier estimate of 128 g protein. We now accept 70 g, and many people are known who can live healthily on far less.

Any estimate, made by even the most competent of dietitians, is to be accepted for the average person only. *No such person exists.* In diet, as in all human affairs, individuality matters. The estimates are statistical, and statistics applied to the single person or event often lie. To take an analogy from physics: we can put a thermometer in a beaker of water and find the temperature is 16.5°C. This is an expression of the average Brownian movement of all the molecules of water in the beaker. Some molecules will be moving at rates corresponding to a far higher temperature and others to a lower temperature. Any individual person is like one of these water molecules. He may not need exactly 70 g of protein each day. He may be able to get by with only 40 g, or he may eat 140 g with no observable damage. This sort of individual variation, which is a stumbling block to the earnest dietitian keen on certainty, may some day be explained, but until that day dietetics (along with much of biology and medicine) can hardly be called an exact science.

One explanation may lie in the efficiency of the digestive system. X's small intestine may absorb a greater percentage of the amino acids in its liver than Y's. Z's liver may produce more bile salts than A's, and so render fat-soluble vitamins in the food more absorbable. M's intestines may contain more bacteria that destroy ascorbic acid or make B-group vitamins than do N's.

Another explanation may be found in the metabolic efficiency of various organs of the body: the circulation, the lungs, endocrine organs, nervous system and muscles. We know that the trained athlete may develop more power from a given muscle mass than the untrained person; that the happy person works better than the neurotic. Perhaps this last observation reveals something about the anecdote concerning Polly, at the beginning of the chapter. It can lead us on to consider the relation between body and mind and its influence upon nutrition.

The influences of the mind upon a person's nutrition

To what extent are the practices of peoples, tribes or nations the result of 'instincts' or of learning and training? How much attention should the dietitian pay to the person's own desires? For example, someone who has been prescribed cod liver oil may either loathe it or like it. Is he to attempt to overcome his loathing, persevere in spite of it, or to acknowledge this loathing as a signal that *his* body does not need that food? If the latter view be accepted it makes dietetics still more lawless and inexact as a science; for it is not only cod liver oil that may be rejected, but such things as green vegetables, wholemeal bread, milk or meat, or even in a patient with anorexia nervosa, the whole idea of eating enough food to maintain life itself.

Opinion divides on this point. One school of dietetic thought maintains that 'instinct' guides the choice of foods. The laboratory rat, deprived for a time of one or another inorganic material, will choose, when allowed, that dish which contains the missing material. Children, so some used to say, take cod liver oil more readily in the winter than in the summer, when sunlight enables them to dispense with a dietary source of cholecalciferol. The sudden whims of a pregnant woman for unusual foods are explained as an instinctual choice of some dietary constituent needed to redress some undetected imbalance in their metabolism, such as excess sugar to prevent an incipient ketosis (see p. 28 on fat metabolism).

The opposite school of thought believes that food habits are brought about by training and upbringing, by external influences such as advertising or chance occurrence with a strong psychological overtone. Much of the rest of this chapter will be concerned with a study of these factors and a critical analysis of instinct in dietary habits.

Conditioning (either in the Pavlovian or Skinnerian sense or more loosely) is notoriously a cause of food fashions. Even mealtimes are conditioned. In a person used to a mid-morning snack, its omission (even if the person is not aware that he has forgotten it) will cause that sinking feeling. If his whole lifestyle has changed, after a few days without the snack, eleven o'clock will pass with no untoward sensations. Similarly, a person used to eating at 1 p.m. who mistakes the 12.45 hooter for the 1 o'clock, will feel hunger as if it were 1 p.m. In the same way are our food choices conditioned by training and habits. Anyone who travels will have noticed that. Bread is a natural article of diet in western civilisation and rice a food that one eats occasionally. In much of South-East Asia, rice is the 'staff of life' and bread an occasional adjunct. The rice-eating Bengali in 1944 preferred to starve to death rather than eat wheat flour (though his descendants in Bangladesh in the 1970s accept wheat readily, thus illustrating the further point that conditioning will change, given time). In South Germany it is customary to serve stewed cherries with roast beef and gooseberry jam with boiled beef—unheard of mixtures in Britain, while the German will not combine strawberries with cream!

What one is brought up to eat, that one eats willingly for the rest of one's life, only rarely venturing upon new foods. It took at least 200 years to popularise the potato and at least 100 years for tomatoes to become accepted in Britain, while bananas and grapefruit each took 30 years from their first introduction. An enormous sales resistance still exists to raw vegetable salads, though they have been eaten in North America since at least the 1920s, and any British country schoolboy, given the chance, will steal a carrot or turnip from a field and eat it raw! Food habits are handed on from generation to generation, and different peoples, even in the same environment, develop very different habits. The place of instinct becomes very doubtful when one considers the almost wholly vegetable diet of the Kikuyu in Kenya in comparison with the milk, meat and blood diet of their neighbouring Masai.

If instinct operates at all, then it is a very poor guide to safe and sound dietetics. Otherwise the numerous nutritional deficiency diseases could not have arisen. Where was the strong instinct for right feeding that allows us to prefer white bread and polished rice? And why did not instinct guide a maritime nation like the English to eat fish livers and so escape rickets (once known as the 'English Disease').

Some food habits in an individual are traceable to some particular event in the person's past that may have had a strong emotional content. Both at home when I was young and later at boarding school, coffee was only served at breakfast on Sundays. I have forever associated coffee with looking forward to a pleasant and relaxed time—even though I now drink it whenever a pause in the day's routine occurs! Many of my strongest dislikes are linked with unhappy school experiences. I am sure that every reader will have similar strong likes and dislikes, for which he or she can clearly remember the origin. There may be others, the origin of which has been forgotten or even, in a Freudian way, suppressed so that they remain as a symbol of some emotional disturbance.

Conditioning of food habits is deliberately used in advertising, and here it is mostly employed in a commercial manner, to encourage the increased consumption of a particular product of a single manufacturer or group. The slogan 'drinka pinta milka day', was designed to raise the level of consumption of one particular valuable food commodity, but similar advertising campaigns can as easily and as effectively be mounted to encourage us to eat any form of food. The 'drinka pinta' campaign began before advertising on television reached a high level of activity. I am sure that this medium and the weekly magazines can between them determine very largely what we want to eat, perhaps by making us think that this is what those people whom we wish to resemble are eating. This sort of advertising is very compelling in its effects and it can be used, perhaps not knowingly, either for good or for ill.

Closely related to conditioned food habits is the undoubted influence of states of the mind upon digestion. The unhappy do not feel hunger and digest their food poorly, whereas the eager and happy person has a good appetite and digestion. It is known that painful emotions slow the flow of digestive secretions and reduces the movements of the gut. Similarly, if the food itself is liked, salivary and gastric secretions increase; if disliked, they fail. While some foods have intrinsically more pleasant flavours than others—especially when the latter are unfamiliar—even those that initially act more as an emetic, may eventually stimulate a great flow of digestive juices. It is likely that the taste for any and every food except mother's milk is acquired, and the production of digestive secretions on seeing, smelling or tasting it is what physiologists call a conditioned reflex response. It is certainly true that every food that a person likes evokes pleasure when eaten and that this pleasure conduces to good digestion. The reverse is also true. Further, pleasing accompaniments to a meal (good service, pleasant surroundings, napery, cutlery etc.) influence digestion favourably and the reverse, unfavourably. Good temper encourages good digestion; bad temper, worry or anxiety result in dyspepsia.

Enough has been said to show that the twin sciences of nutrition and dietetics can never be as accurate as physics or chemistry, and that great accuracy may not always be needed, possible or worthwhile—so varied is the physiological behaviour of different people. When psychology intervenes, or the altered physiology of little understood disease states, all certainty, and rational prediction vanish—as in the case of Polly.

The main deductions of this chapter so far are (1) that it is impossible to be exact about diet and dietetics because of the variations in foods and in peoples. (2) Consequently the best devised schemes of diet may produce no results when applied to the individual though they may be good in the mass. (3) The practising dietitian must carry these facts in mind and learn to work within the limits they set, and also remember (4) that an optimal diet alone is not enough for a good life. It must be accompanied by the other conditions of housing etc. needed for its enjoyment.

Nutritional planning

None the less, there is no need to despair about dietetics. It cannot be an exact science and it may fail utterly with some individuals, but that it has been, is, and increasingly will be a great help to both the single person and the community cannot be doubted. The guidance of British government policy in the 1939–45 war by dietitians not only ensured the satisfactory health of the people but an actual improvement in health beyond all previous standards. Food manufacturers, guided by dietetic discoveries, put foods on the market which combined a pleasant taste with dietetic value, e.g. blackcurrant purée, concentrated orange juice and rose-hip syrup, all of which replaced the unavailable citrus fruit as sources of ascorbic acid.

Although it really belongs to the next chapter on building an optimal diet, more will be said here about ways of improving people's diets. Apart from political and economic considerations, there are also physiological and psychological ones to be remembered. There are short-term and long-term solutions also.

In the short-term we work within the restrictions imposed by existing food likes and dislikes, or alter them by slow and gradual means. For example, a person is told that cod liver oil would improve his health, but it nauseates him and he cannot learn a conditioned taste for it. Capsules of the oil may help, but they are expensive, difficult for some to swallow and the flavour may still regurgitate from stomach or oesophagus. The other foods containing retinol and cholecalciferol are the fat fish (herrings, bloaters, kippers, sprats, whitebait, sardines, salmon and mackerel) and it may be that our person will eat sufficient of one of these. The quantity of these foods equivalent to one teaspoonful of cod liver oil may, however be quite large, expensive and scarce. Anyway, he may not like these, but will eat the

12
The optimal diet

It is now possible to summarise the facts and recommendations put down in the preceding chapters and to show, briefly, how an *optimal diet* may be built up. By 'optimal diet' I mean the best possible diet. This is not the most expensive diet, or the cheapest. It is not the most varied or the most monotonous, nor the most original or conventional, the most or the least convenient diet. It is that diet that *cannot be improved* by the addition of any other constituent. Furthermore, there must be many hundreds of optimal diets.

If man were a rigid machine there could be but one optimal diet, containing so many grams of purified amino acids, carbohydrates, fats, vitamins and inorganic materials. But man is not a standard, production-line product. His energy and other needs vary from person to person. Even if he were standardised, it would matter little to his body whether he obtained his amino acids from meat, milk or vegetable proteins, his thiamine from bacon or bran, his iron from liver or from black treacle. Dietitians must be ready to vary their choice of optimal diets to suit individual and cultural preferences, and to work within limits set by climate and season and by economic necessity.

The optimal diet must be determined both by the objective, scientific point of view, and from the practical, personal and economic standpoints. The scientist says that a diet must contain so much protein, yield so many joules and have so many milligrams of the various inorganic materials and vitamins available. The amounts will depend upon age, sex and occupation of the recipient. In the previous chapters, under each factor, estimates of these amounts have been given. In Table 12.1 are summarised many of the British Department of Health and Social Security recommendations of 1969. This table looks pretty formidable but it should be remembered that this is a *tentative* goal only, the aim when planning practical dietaries, to be approached through a good diet of natural foods. It is no hard and fast law to be met in every detail on every day, but should be considered as a standard against which we can measure the values of given diets and improve these should they need improvement. In some respects, as has already been described, the recommendations have erred on the side of safety, and are more generous than necessary. This applies perhaps to ascorbic acid, to calcium, and even to protein. Cholecalciferol may not be needed at all in the food if exposure to natural sunlight is generous.

Table 12.1 The DHSS recommended daily dietary intakes (1969).

	Body weight	Energy	Protein	Thiamine	Riboflavin	Nicotinic acid	Ascorbic acid	Retinol	Cholecalciferol	Calcium	Iron
	kg	MJ	g	g	mg	mg	mg	μg	μg	mg	mg
Children											
0–1	7.3	3.3	20	0.3	0.4	5	15	450	10.0	600	6
1–3	12.5	5.5	28	0.6	0.7	8	20	300	10.0	500	7
3–5	16.5	6.7	40	0.6	0.8	9	20	300	10.0	500	8
5–9	22.8	8.2	49	0.8	1.0	11	20	400	2.5	500	9
Boys											
9–12	31.9	10.5	63	1.0	1.2	14	25	575	2.5	700	13
12–15	45.5	11.7	70	1.1	1.4	16	25	725	2.5	600	15
15–18	61.0	12.6	75	1.2	1.7	19	30	750	2.5	600	15
Girls											
9–12	33.0	9.6	58	0.9	1.2	13	25	575	2.5	700	13
12–15	48.6	9.6	58	0.9	1.4	16	25	725	2.5	700	14
15–18	56.1	9.6	58	0.9	1.4	16	30	750	2.5	600	15
Men											
Sedentary	65	11.1	67	1.1	1.7	18	30	750	2.5	500	10
Active	65	12.4	74	1.2	1.7	18	30	750	2.5	500	10
Retired	63	9.3	57	0.9	1.7	18	30	750	2.5	500	10
Women											
Sedentary	55	9.2	55	0.9	1.3	15	30	750	2.5	500	12
Active	55	10.5	63	1.0	1.3	15	30	750	2.5	500	12
Pregnant (4–9 months)		10.0	60	1.0	1.6	18	60	750	10.0	1200	15
Lactation		11.3	68	1.1	1.8	21	60	1200	10.0	1200	15
Retired		8.3	50	0.8	1.3	15	30	750	2.5	500	10

Planning the optimal diet

There are two ways of tackling the problem of getting an optimal diet. One is to take an actual diet, critically examine it along with Table 12.1 and by altering it, bring it up to the recommendations. The other is to start from the table and build up a diet from scratch. The first is the traditional British way of solving the problem—the empirical way—but the latter is the more rational, scientific or radical method. Each will eventually achieve the same result.

For either method we need to group foods according to their functions. This has been attempted in detail in Chapters 5, 7, 8 and 9. It would be helpful to summarise the information here.

Foods for energy

Dripping, frying fats, suet, butter, margarine, bacon, cheese, flour, bread, cakes, biscuits, sugar, jam, dried fruits, potatoes.

Foods for proteins

Milk, cheese, meat, fish, eggs, grain *and* pulses (taken together).

Foods for inorganic materials

Calcium: Cheese, fat fish, milk, eggs.
Iron: Liver, meat, eggs, green vegetables.
Iodine: Sea fish, seaweeds.

Foods for vitamins

Retinol: Dairy foods, margarine, green and yellow vegetables, liver.
Cholecalciferol: Fish liver oils, fat fish, summer milk and butter, margarine.
Thiamine: Yeast, wheat germ, liver, kidneys, pig meat, whole cereals.
Riboflavine: Yeast, wheat germ, liver, meat, fish, eggs, cheese.
Nicotinic acid: Yeast, wheat germ and bran, liver and kidneys, meat (but any tryptophan-rich protein will do).
Ascorbic acid: Summer fruits, citrus fruits, tomatoes, green vegetables, liver, potatoes.

If we leave aside for the moment energy and protein needs, but pay attention to the foods containing inorganic materials and vitamins, we can group these roughly as follows:

(1) Dairy foods, i.e. milk, butter, cheese and eggs, margarine.
(2) Greengroceries, i.e. green vegetables, carrots, tomatoes, summer and citrus fruits.
(3) Sea produce, the fish liver oils, fat fish, other fish and seaweeds.
(4) Whole-grain cereals.
(5) Liver and other offals.

These foods are collectively called *protective foods*. The term originated in their ability to protect rats from the harmful effects of an exclusively cereal diet. The term has since been widened to include all foods containing vitamins and inorganic materials in significant amounts.

It is easy to criticise the term. It is qualitative, and is not really descriptive. All foods protect against hunger and death in 50 days. Water protects against death in 4 days. The body can carry on for months with a deficient intake of calcium, iron, iodine, retinol, cholecalciferol or ascorbic acid. Furthermore the term has been abused. Foods have been described as 'protected' when their vitamins have not been removed by milling, processing or cooking. The best use of the term is to include in its scope all foods that protect the lay person from being, dietetically, a fool. The term, in this sense, is useful for educational purposes. It is because the diet in Britain, especially if the affluent days of the 1960s and early 1970s really do not return again, as well as that of most other people throughout the world, really does need improvement by the addition of just these foods listed above, that the term should be retained. As was stated earlier (Chapter 2, p. 11), an increase of 60–100% in the production and consumption of protective foods is needed, to make the British diet optimal. If farmers, politicians, economists and businessmen can be roused to action by the term 'protective foods', then that will be justification for its use.

Getting down to details

Given a diet: is it good or bad, and, if bad, how is it to be improved? A dietitian may be presented with a set of menus for criticism and suggestions. I have used a summary of a typical day's food intake several times in earlier chapters of this book.

The following one comes from a residential school:

Breakfast: Porridge, bacon, ½ fried tomato, bread and butter, jam, tea.
Mid-morning: 250 ml milk
Dinner: Cold roast beef, mashed potatoes, pickles, rice pudding.
Tea: Brown and white bread and butter, small cake or scone, tea.
Supper: Brown and white bread and butter, baked beans on toast, water.

It represents a single day's meals, and would probably be found to be repeated on the same day of the week, term by term! First of all we cannot say much about such a set of meals until we know the quantities served and consumed, and about the rest of the week's meals. However, some valuable criticisms and suggestions can be made, even upon such meagre evidence, by applying the list of protective foods to the menus.

The dairy foods are represented by milk and butter only. If a pint of milk had been consumed, the diet would be passed on that score. But cheese is completely neglected on the sample day and, as a matter of fact, on every other day of the week, also. This is a senseless and a serious omission. Green and salad vegetables and the protective fruits are also absent, except for half a tomato. The pickles could be replaced with a salad containing tomatoes, watercress, mustard and cress, radishes, raw cabbage etc. Or if they were replaced by carrots, then an orange or *real* lemonade could be given later in the day, or some fresh, frozen or tinned summer fruits (it is possible that an institution such as the one providing this material has its own gardens, where the fruits and vegetables could be grown on the premises).

The remaining groups of protective foods similarly are not present in this specimen menu. Some of the bread, admittedly, is brown, but the fortified white bread does not replace all the components of wholemeal bread. Fat fish, fish liver oils, and meat offals need to be brought into the diet. They appeared nowhere in the whole week. Instead of the baked beans, herrings, mackerel or fish roe might well appear, or a white fish cooked in a white sauce fortified with cod liver oil. One or two such meals a week would be ample. And the offal? Kidneys, except beef kidneys (which cost no more than a shin of beef) are expensive, many people do not like heart or liver when served in a *recognisable* form, and pig's liver is likely to be tough. But both heart and liver form the basis of excellent patés (which can be made long before the meal at which they are eaten, to the caterer's delight!) There are also the savoury (but supposedly vulgar) dishes of haggis, faggots and tripe, all of which should be considered by a dietetically-minded caterer.

In this way, most 'middle-class' diets (which are normally adequate in energy and animal protein) can easily be made wholly satisfactory, by replacing some of the foods served with alternatives drawn from the lists of protective foods. All varieties of the latter should be well represented. Such a method of building up an optimal diet involves but the simplest knowledge of dietetics and, moreover, it avoids any narrow-minded fanaticisms which, though they solve one problem, ignore or compound others.

The radical way of producing an optimal diet

In the past there have been sundry dietetic parodies of the proverb, 'look after the pence, and the pounds will look after themselves'. During the 1914–18 war, one such was, 'look after the calories (energy), and the proteins will look after themselves'. In writing earlier chapters of this book, I have been tempted to say 'look after the amino acids and the B-complex of vitamins will look after themselves'. But this immediately shows the danger of such slogans. I have left out ascorbic acid, the fat-soluble vitamins and calcium. While simple appetite or hunger will look after energy, they will do no more and no simple aphorism will sum up all we ought to do in dietetics. The best is: *Take care of the protective foods; make up any deficit that remains in protein of high biological value, and then let appetite look after energy*. To that should be added a couple of cautions: maintain body weight at the life insurance table figures for 25 years old, and remember that saturated fats *may* prove to be harmful to arteries.

Unguided choice will never lead a child or adult human to the right foods. Apples and plums are just as pleasant to eat as blackcurrants or strawberries, but are devoid of ascorbic acid. Choice is so completely conditioned by upbringing and social pressures that we can never rely on it. We are not rats who may deliberately select salty rather than pure water to drink when they are salt-depleted. Nor are we like the group of North American babies, 6–18 months old, who were allowed 'unlimited' choice over what and how much they ate. All throve and this has been held to show that they had instinctively chosen the right foods. *This is not so.* All the foods offered belonged to the protective foods, the babies not being given white bread, sugar or sweets etc. No doubt, it would be to everyone's advantage if we could live on protective foods only. Unfortunately we cannot afford to do so, for they cost too much. We must, in planning our diet, provide enough of the protective foods to ensure we have the recommended amounts of essential nutrients and then fill in the gaps left in energy, rather than use the protective foods as our diet, or use them only when hunger has been satisfied (which is what the world's, and Britain's, poor are forced to do). A reasonable start on a daily allowance of protective foods is shown in Table 12.2. When the yields of these are calculated the results as shown in Table 12.3. are found.

Table 12.2 The daily protective foods content of an optimal diet.

Dairy produce		Greengroceries		Fish		Cereals
Milk	0.5l	Tomatoes	120g	Herring	60g	Fortified bread or
Cheese	30g	Greens or				wholemeal bread 200g
Butter or		carrots	120g			
margarine	45g					
Egg	50g					

Before going any further some comments must be made on Table 12.3. First, a criticism I regularly make of students' work in physiology, is that many of these values are given to four significant figures. If they mean anything at all, it is only the second, or possibly the third figure that should be considered. Thus 1271 should be 1300, 8.47 as 8.5, 1129 as 1100 and so on. Second, though there is a general resemblance between these figures and those in earlier editions of this book, there are some changes. Retinol and cholecalciferol are named and the quantities are given in micrograms; no longer do we refer to vitamin A or D or to I.U. (international units). Third, note again that, in order to obtain anything near a sufficiency of the required materials, a mixed diet is essential. Our calcium comes from milk, cheese and bread, iron from egg and bread (though it is unlikely that the finely-divided metallic iron, added to bread by government order, is absorbed), retinol from dairy produce and greens, ascorbic acid from tomatoes and greens and cholecalciferol from the herring.

Is this diet, chosen entirely from the protective foods, enough? In addition to the values given in Table 12.3 for inorganic materials and vitamins, the diet contains 66 g protein, of which 43 g are of high biological value—more than the minimum recommended. It has 90 g fat, but only 150 g carbohydrate and its energy value is only 6.11 MJ: obviously not enough. While it has enough calcium, retinol and ascorbic acid, it is low for iron, the B vitamins and perhaps cholecalciferol. We need these and another 4–6 MJ.

Table 12.3 The amounts of essential nutrients obtained from the protective foods listed in Table 12.2.

		Calcium mg	Iron mg	Retinol μg	Cholecalciferol μg	Thiamine mg	Riboflavine mg	Nicotinic acid mg	Ascorbic acid mg
Milk	0.5l	680	0.40	255	0.21	0.23	0.85	0.45	11.3
Cheese	30g	230	0.16	119	0.10	0.01	0.14	0.03	nil
Butter	45g	6	0.07	387	0.43	nil	nil	nil	nil
Egg	50g	32	1.48	170	2.43	0.86	0.20	0.40	nil
Tomatoes	120g	15	0.48	48	nil	0.07	0.05	0.78	22.7
Greens	120g	34	0.80	120	nil	0.07	0.06	0.28	68.1
Herring	60g	66	0.98	30	14.40	0.02	0.19	2.27	nil
Bread	200g	208	4.10	nil	nil	0.41	nil	3.86	nil
Totals		1271	8.47	1129	17.57	0.86	1.49	8.07	102.1

Very few people would be satisfied with the meat content of this diet, so we should add 50 g bacon and 50 g of meat per day. The diet now has 12 mg iron, 1.1 mg thiamine, 1.7 mg riboflavine and 12 mg nicotinic acid. Apart from this last, all are now satisfactory, and the tryptophan content of meat and milk will satisfy the nicotinic acids needs. The total energy content has been raised by 1.2 MJ approx. The only gap remaining is that of energy. This can be filled in any way that is agreeable, convenient or economic. The wealthy would eat more butter and meat. Potatoes might be added, or jam etc. eaten with bread and butter. Cream and sweets or pastries are great providers of energy. Sugars and alcohol—especially spirits—can add energy to the diet, though nothing else. A 'middle class' diet would certainly have still more meat and fish and fresh fruit and salads. There should be no difficulty in making the diet completely satisfactory—even by North American standards—by a wise choice among the foods taken to make up the energy deficit.

This example is not intended as any sort of universal prescription for an optimal diet, but only as an indication of the way to plan such a diet. There are thousands of possible optimal diets, any of which can be reached by starting from the following principles:

(1) Make sure of inorganic materials and vitamins from the protective foods.
(2) Then check that the protein of high biological value is adequate.
(3) Finally make up, *but do not exceed*, the deficit in energy.

Unfortunately, all poor people work the other way round. They go for energy first. Cheap foods supply energy and little else—for sources of good protein, vitamins and the inorganic materials are expensive. Hence in two-thirds or more of the human race are found malnourishment, stunted growth, a short expectation of life, and diseases such as anaemia, kwashiorkor, xerophthalmia, beri-beri, pellagra, scurvy and rickets or osteomalacia.

13
Practical dietetics

So far we have dealt with some of the basic theories and facts of nutrition and foods, as well as some of the equally theoretical problems incurred when attempting to relate these theories and facts to actual dietaries. The word 'dietary' originally meant 'a way of daily life', or what a person did with his day. Today, the simpler word 'diet' means a person's food intake, but one should always remember that this must be seen in relation to his whole daily way of life. In this chapter we will study diets in relation to dietaries and see how diets should be modified to meet any particular condition of life in which a person might find himself.

As has been stated many times already, a dietary standard is more an indication than a rule. It may, and should, apply to the mass of people, and be true *on average*, but it does not have to apply to each single person. The best-laid schemes of diet often fail because of individual peculiarities or idiosyncrasies, as described in Chapter 11.

How many meals a day?

The practical answers to this have been many and have varied according to the country and the century. The English eat a large breakfast, in France a small one is the rule, whereas in Holland cold meats and cheese appear at breakfast! The African labourer in Johannesburg has adopted (or has been persuaded to accept) a working day with no meal break and then a large evening meal.

Custom has similarly crystallised in North America and Australia into a 3-meal daily regime. In Britain it is three and at least one small snack. Among the wealthy one finds places for three main meals and four snacks! (Early morning tea and biscuit, breakfast, 'elevenses', lunch, afternoon tea, dinner and finally a snack with the whisky night-cap.) The times of the main meals has also changed considerably over the years. Anyone who reads Jane Austin's novels will immediately be aware of this. Then there is the practice of the 2–4 hour siesta in many hot countries. Such diversity in practice suggests that no physiologically determined rule exists. There is only the anatomical determinant—our stomachs are not large enough to contain at one time the sheer bulk of food needed each day.

Studies have been made of muscular efficiency (mechanical work output ÷ sum of work output and heat output) before breakfast and later in the day. Efficiency is at its *lowest* before breakfast, reaches a peak about an hour after breakfast and then falls again. Further peaks occur after lunch and the evening meal. If additional smaller meals are introduced in the morning and afternoon, further subsidiary peaks in efficiency are observed. These studies were originally made on trained laboratory staff, working on a stationary bicycle ergometer. They were also found to be true for school teachers and children. Finally, similar tests were made on factory workers. Not only was efficiency adversely affected by missing a meal, but absenteeism was commoner both among those who habitually missed meals and in the test groups who were asked to forgo meals as part of the studies on muscular efficiency. Conversely, absenteeism was less among workers who casually ate between meals, as the spirit moved them.

There seemed little doubt in the results of these studies. It is better to take regular meals than to miss a meal at a time when one is accustomed to eating. Further studies showed that it was better still, from the point of view of muscular efficiency, to take five meals (mid-morning and mid-afternoon snacks) in the working day than three. The only argument raised against this last is that a person is thereby putting more food into his stomach before the previous meal has wholly left it. The stomach therefore 'gets no rest'. But why should it rest? The heart, kidneys and lungs never rest, nor does the small intestine. 'Resting' the stomach is the sort of rule, evolved out of some inner consciousness and based on no physiological evidence, that has bemused dietitians ever since man began thinking about food. Moreover, it may even be harmful, for gastric juice undiluted by food is more likely to cause indigestion and ulcers than when mixed with more food. Peptic ulcer patients may, indeed, do better on a 'little and often' regime or even on a continuous intra-gastric milk drip, fashionable when I was a medical student.

The authors of these studies made one very important point. They suggested that the snacks should consist mainly of protective foods. They feared that if energy foods were eaten then, the total protective food content of the day's diet might be too low (today we might worry that the energy content is too high!) The snacks should consist of a banana (for ascorbic acid) a glass of milk, or cress, tomato or sardine sandwich, rather than sweet coffee and biscuits, sugary soft drinks or sweet buns.

Regularity of meals

It is usual to inculcate regularity as being of the greatest importance. But one should ask: to whom is it important? In business it matters to the workship or office manager, to the cook and to the caterer. It might help the individual to establish regular conditioned reflexes to fit in with regular work routines. But if the work schedule is essentially irregular, then such conditioning may be a nuisance. Some people have a glucose-regulating system that allows excessive falls of blood glucose levels 3–4 hours after the last meal, when they become increasingly inefficient, both physically and mentally. For them, as for those with regular routines, it is best to adopt the inevitable and arrange for mealtimes to occur at preordained times. We have already seen that those who are careless about eating between meals are less often absent from work than the meticulous, and it is likely that the happy-go-lucky person who doesn't worry about mealtimes is better off than the one who keeps rigidly to a set schedule and gets very anxious when his schedule is upset. Such a person will worry himself into indigestion (or worse) if this happens too often.

Drinking at meals

It has been argued, again without factual evidence, that drinks with meals delay digestion because they dilute the gastric juice. Some will even adopt a rigorous rule of no drinks with meals. It should be pointed out that (i) even if dilution does slow digestion it will probably slow it in proportion to the square root of the degree of dilution. Halving the concentration of an enzyme reduces its rate of reaction to $1/\sqrt{2}$ or to 70% of its original rate and dilution to 1 in 3 slows the rate to 58%; (ii) water is a gentle stimulus to secretion; (iii) finally, a meal that is enjoyed calls forth more gastric juice than one that is not liked. From all these theoretical arguments on the other side it looks as though the ordinary person may drink with meals. After all, this has been the practice for some thousands of years without harm.

There are two groups of people who should perhaps modify this common custom. A 'sloppy' meal leaves the stomach more slowly than a dry one. A sluggish stomach (diagnosed by a competent physician backed up with X-ray examination) may be helped therefore by reducing the fluids at mealtimes, while an overactive one may be helped with copious fluids.

Rest and meals

There is no doubt that exercise, particularly that which uses the abdominal muscles is good for digestion. It is perhaps in part due to the massage of the gut stimulating it to motor activity, but it is more likely the result of a general feeling of well-being that exercise induces. Vigorous activity results in a redistribution of circulating blood, to muscles and to skin, and away from the gut. Secretion and motility of the stomach decrease in heavy exercise, the food being less well digested and mixed, and gastric emptying is delayed. It is therefore usually suggested that no vigorous exercise be taken for 30–60 minutes after a large meal. Some advocate a period of rest before meals, but I can see no reason for this. In many private-sector schools such a rest-period after the midday meal used to be regularly prescribed, and according to the headmasters, with benefit. If it was good for the cream of the adolescent life, it is probably good for all! It gives the opportunity for the full neural secretion of gastric juice (p. 24), after which affairs can be left to themselves.

'Bowel regularity'

It used to be believed, and still is dwindlingly in patent medicine advertising, that the large intestinal contents should be kept regularly on the move, if necessary with all sorts of medicinal purgatives or laxative substances. It was thought that stasis caused the production and absorption of poisonous 'amines' from non-absorbed amino acids. The fashion of the 1970s is that colonic contents are best kept soft and bulky, and so regularly and easily moved forwards by eating foods containing 'fibre'. This is a bad term, for not all compounds included in 'fibre' are fibrous. They are non-digestible and therefore non-absorbable materials, are mostly polysaccharides of various types, such as cellulose from plant cell walls, agar from seaweeds, pecten from fruits, and guar gum, obtained from the cluster bean. All these compounds increase the bulk of the colonic content, and render it softer. The bulk increase stimulates more activity of the muscle and the softness of the material enhances the effectiveness of muscle contraction. People whose diet has a high 'fibre' content seem to suffer less from diverticular disease of the colon, and less from haemorrhoids than others, but the cause-effect link between the nature of colonic contents and these two diseases has not been experimentally established. A high 'fibre' diet may also be beneficial in that it may slow the rate of glucose and fat absorption from the small gut, and thus reduce the liability to develop diabetes and arterial disease. One causative factor in both diseases may be the rate of rise in blood glucose and fat concentrations respectively in the absorptive period after eating.

The next part of this chapter will be concerned with special dietary provisions that should be made for various age-groups of healthy people, and for people living under different work and environmental conditions.

Infant nutrition

The feeding of the very young is a matter for dietitians when healthy babies are concerned, and for co-operative work with paediatricians when sickness intervenes. This specialised area of nutrition is, of necessity, more empirical than scientific. Except where conditions are already very abnormal, it is unusual for the research worker to be able to perform controlled experiments and modify the nutrition of infants, in the way that this can be done with adults whose 'informed consent' can readily be obtained. Moreover, our ideas about infant nutrition change frequently and rapidly. Nonetheless there are some attitudes and practices that are worth discussing. Paediatricians are still concerned that, if it can be in any way managed, breast feeding is the best way of feeding a baby. Human milk was evolved through biological processes over millions of years to be the best possible food for human infants, and the infants' digestive and other systems have similarly evolved to live on human milk. If, for any medical, social or economic reason it is impossible for the baby to be reared at the breast, his best chance of survival depends on being given food that imitates, as nearly as possible, both in quantity and quality, that which he would otherwise be receiving. Of other mammalian milks, cow's milk is by far the most freely available in Britain and most parts of the world. It contains more protein (3.3%, compared with 1.2%), but less sugar and fat than human milk. The energy contents of the two are almost the same. Human milk contains more retinol, nicotinic acid and ascorbic acid, but less thiamine and riboflavine. The conspicuous difference that matters in many climates is the high content of salt in cow's milk, over three times that of human milk. While a moderate intake of salts, as seen in Chapter 8, is essential, excesses have to be excreted in the urine and require water for this excretion. An infant on cow's milk is more liable to suffer from water shortage than one at the breast. Cow's milk also contains more phosphate than human milk, and it may be that this, when absorbed into the infant's body fluids, causes a harmful reduction in both calcium and magnesium levels.

The high protein content of cow's milk is not well tolerated by some infants due to tough casein curd formation, though preliminary boiling of the liquid milk avoids this. To overcome the other problems, the simplest solution has been to dilute the cow's milk with an equal volume of water, to which sufficient sucrose is added to restore the total energy content of the milk. It has now become the custom to prepare dried milk powders from liquid cow's milk which can be modified to suit human infants. In these the salt, phosphate, protein and vitamin concentrations can be adjusted to be optimal for human infant's needs. If these products are used, then precise instructions for their use, *which can be understood and followed by those preparing the foods*, must also be supplied. Much expense, ingenuity and sales promotion has gone into the marketing of these materials and while they may be life saving or a great convenience if properly used, their misuse can lead to individual and social disasters. While it is difficult to kill babies, one should remember that 'light of nature', 'maternal instinct', or even 'plain commonsense' are poor substitutes for rational understanding of the requirements of the human infant, and when difficulties arise the expert in this understanding should be at hand. When the writer was at the breast and bottle stage in the 1920s the rule was to stick to a rigid timetable: meals every 3 hours for a tiny baby and every 4 hours for a strong and healthy baby. No matter how much he yelled, food was withheld until the correct time. That practice was being gradually relaxed when the first edition of this book was published, and the idea that babies should be fed 'on demand' was gaining ground. Infants were held to know best when they wanted food and if they howled they were to be fed. This theory still holds, but the practice is rarely carried out after the first baby of a family, as one might expect! No one knows what either the physiological or psychological effects of rigid adherence to either set of rules may be, but one must remember how easily a person can become conditioned to set mealtimes.

The feeding of solid foods, it is now recommended (Oppé *et al.*, 1974), should not commence before 4 months of age. Cereal products should also not be added to bottle feeds. The reasons given for these proscriptions are first that there is no evidence of an advantage in the infant's health and development when cereal or other foods are provided at an earlier age, and secondly, that sensitivity to gluten, a wheat protein associated with coeliac disease, may develop if this is given early in life.

Initially, the solids are provided as purées or, in the case of cereal products, as powders which are easily converted to a soft paste by the addition of milk or water. No person takes automatically to new textures and flavours, so it is necessary to lead the infant on from one already-accepted flavour to others by judicious mixtures. Ascorbic acid rich fruit juices or purées are one useful starting point. Puréed liver is another very useful one, for it provides iron at a time when the iron stores bequeathed by the mother before birth may be running low. During this period, also, the salt content of foods may be too high and lead to excessive water loss. Extra salt, to suit parental tastes, should *not* be added to infants' foods.

Obesity in infants is now relatively common, though it is beyond the scope of this book to define the ideal weight for age of infants, or their weight-for-length relationship. Nonetheless such standards exist and both immediate and long-term problems may occur in those who greatly exceed these ideals. As in adults, an excess of intake over requirement inevitably results in obesity, and the cure is to reduce intake. Once babies become mobile, activity raises requirement and the problem may cure itself, though some people assert that obese infants become obese adults, through a profound and life-long alteration of their metabolic processes.

Diet in adolescence

At the onset of puberty, in both sexes, appetite increases with the increase in growth rate and accompanies the increase seen in daily energy expenditure (which is, of course, reflected by the rise in daily food intake). Appetite, though, is the desire to eat, not just the process of eating and the increase in appetite in adolescence may result in many new foods being accepted and enjoyed, as well as larger amounts of the accustomed staples.

Since bone and muscle growth, particularly in boys, are the dominant feature of the adolescent growth spurt, foods containing calcium and protein of high biological value should be given in larger amounts at this time. Milk and cheese are particularly valuable and no adolescent should be told that only babies or cissies drink milk, or now that he is growing up he should change to tea, coffee or beer. Girls at puberty should be encouraged to eat more of the iron-rich foods, since their iron losses are becoming, due to menstruation, larger than boys'. Liver, meat, greens and eggs should feature regularly in their food.

It must be remembered in institutional catering that the 14–21-year-olds cannot, for the above reasons, be treated like the average adult. This is, as was described earlier (p. 121), a period when new foods will be avidly accepted, and it is far better for these to be cheese and watercress sandwiches and milk rather than fish, chips and beer! If girls are worried about their weight, they must be encouraged to cut down on cakes, puddings and sweets rather than any of the protective foods.

Diet for the worker

It used to be necessary to see that those whose work demanded a large energy expenditure had an energy intake in their food sufficient to meet these demands. We now have to ensure that the energy intake of the sedentary does not exceed their energy needs. When energy requirements, due to physical activity at work are high, though, there is little increase in urinary nitrogen excretion, indicating that there is little increase in protein breakdown, and that no increase in dietary protein is required. This, of course, flatly contradicts the popular notion that those who do hard muscular work need more protein.

A distinct case exists for raising the thiamine, riboflavine and nicotinic acid intake of people whose work is energetic. The requirements of these vitamins is directly related to the person's energy turnover. Foods, such as wholemeal bread, which supply both energy and these vitamins, are all that is needed for the heavy manual worker. It's his wife who needs the meat, to ensure an adequate iron intake!

Since, as was mentioned earlier, exercise is good for digestion, sedentary work often makes for a poor digestion, and if this work carries any degree of psychological stress, then downright bad digestion and even peptic ulceration may develop. The sedentary person's meals should therefore be small and bland in nature. No special care need be taken if his work is mental. Bertie Wooster may have believed that Jeeves' great mental powers were due to his high consumption of fish, but the resting brain needs the same amounts of the same material (glucose) as that of the most active thinker.

The athlete's diet

Most of the very disparate ideas traditionally held by atheletes and their trainers about the correct dietary for athletes are not related to scientific knowledge of bodily function, and the theories of the dietitians have for long been at variance with the practice of the trainer, but latterly considerable rapprochement has occurred.

An increase in muscle bulk or in intrinsic muscle strength may occur in training regimes. Both require some extra protein, but not in the vast amounts once consumed by Oxford and Cambridge rowing men. The other important factor is a generous supply of oxidisable material at the time of the athletic performance. This means glycogen (for we all have, all the time, such adequate stores of fat around the body that we need not be concerned about their nutritional maintenance in athletics). The glycogen present in muscle is used in short-lasting and explosive events (throwing, jumping and sprinting). That present in the liver is needed, along with fat, for the endurance types of exercise. Both muscle and liver glycogen stores can be somewhat increased by a few days of a high carbohydrate diet, and the liver store may be supplemented by eating glucose during a long-term bout of exercise, such as a championship tennis match. As with the manual workers, if the athelete's regular daily energy expenditure is raised, his intake of B vitamins must be similarly raised, to maintain a constant vitamin:energy ratio.

Vegetarianism has had a vogue among athletes: Finnish long-distance runners and British long-distance cyclists being two examples. So long as milk, eggs and cheese can meet the protein needs, a vegetarian diet may be satisfactory, but a fruit, vegetable and cereal diet is a windy diet and flatulence is a bugbear in athletics.

The average woman's diet

Dietetically speaking, man and woman are different animals. Adolescence begins earlier in girls than in boys, so the nutritional adjustments needed to cater for the growth spurt must be made in time. Thereafter, although she needs the extra iron intake required to cover menstrual iron loss, her needs for proteins, vitamins and energy are less than a man's. Man is a high-geared, high-octane type of engine, capable of great bursts of energy output from his larger muscles. Weight for weight his basal metabolism is also some 10% higher than that of a woman. He needs more energy, therefore, in proportion to the rest of his food. A woman needs less fuel, for her organism is geared to a lower but more prolonged output of work. Her average energy needs are 9.2 MJ/day, though they may exceed 10.5 for a large and active woman. Even a sedentary man needs 11.1 MJ/day, but very active men may need over 15 MJ. Finally, it seems that if dietary energy intake exceeds needs, women are more liable than men to convert the excess to fat (while men burn it off in conspicuous waste!). A woman's food should, therefore, be more heavily weighted, as has already been said for the adolescent girl, towards the protective foods and away from those that supply only energy.

Diet in pregnancy

It is obvious that the diet in pregnancy must be different from that of the non-pregnant woman. Further, she is not just a woman and a fetus, and we must move away from the rather too precise mathematical calculations of the needs of pregnancy, towards general recommendations for an improvement in diet throughout pregnancy, with special emphasis on the protective foods. However, one must have guide-lines and both the Department of Health and Social Services in Great Britain and the American National Academy of Sciences have published their separate, and somewhat different lists of recommendations. The more significant of these are shown in Table 13.1. The DHSS requirements, furthermore, are only to be applied in the latter two-thirds of pregnancy. While the Americans think protein and iron are of outstanding importance, in Britain we emphasise particularly ascorbic acid, cholecalciferol and calcium, though for these we accept a lower intake for the non-pregnant, while advising the same intake as the Americans for the pregnant! These discrepancies, and the illogicality of starting the supplements in Britain only after three months make me incline to the view I have expressed above, that the recommendations are too precise. They are liable to make the pregnant woman over-anxious lest she and the fetus be missing some essential nutrient, or she will say 'it's all too difficult', bury her head in the sand and do nothing at all about it, to her

Table 13.1 Recommended dietary intakes in pregnancy, compared with those of corresponding non-pregnant women.

		British (DHSS, 1969)			American (NAS, 1974)		
		Non-pregnant	Pregnant	% rise	Non-pregnant	Pregnant	% rise
Energy	(MJ)	9.2	10.0	9	8.8	10.1	14
Protein	(g)	55	60	9	46	76	62
Thiamine	(mg)	1.0	1.0	11	1.1	1.4	27
Riboflavin	(mg)	1.3	1.6	23	1.4	1.7	22
Nicotinic acid	(mg)	15	18	20	14	16	14
Ascorbic acid	(mg)	30	60	100	45	60	33
Retinol	(μg)	750	750	nil	800	1000	25
Cholecalciferol	(μg)	2.5	10.0	300	10.0	10.0	nil
Calcium	(mg)	500	1200	140	800	1200	50
Iron	(mg)	12	15	25	18	18*	?

* The NAS recommends that as no diet gives enough iron, supplementary medication must be supplied.

own and her child's ultimate detriment. A simpler and more reasonable, if less rigidly scientific, way to put it is that *from the first* special attempts should be made to increase the *proportions of all protective foods* in the diet, while maintaining a reasonable level of carbohydrate intake in the first three months (nausea is common then, is exacerbated by ketosis, which is reduced by carbohydrates), and adjusting energy intake to ensure an optimal weight gain. Calcium and cholecalciferol intake should be raised after the fourth month, for bone deposition in the fetus begins then. A large transfer of iron from mother to fetus occurs in the last three months and should be balanced by an adequate iron intake (though much may come from iron stores which will then need replenishment).

There is sufficient evidence, amounting almost to scientific proof, that improvement in the diet of pregnant women is of great advantage to mother and baby, and therefore to the whole country. It has been found that good feeding with protective foods lowered maternal and perinatal mortality. While such studies are usually done on those frankly depressed economically, similar results will always be found when the diet is less than optimal. It is noteworthy that with almost everything else against them, maternal mortality, puerperal complications, stillbirths, neonatal and infantile mortality fell markedly in Britain during the 1939–45 war, and since then have fallen still lower. The social classes among whom these were highest prior to 1940 were those who benefited the most, due to their generally improved economic state and to the cheap milk etc. and priority of supply of other protective foods. The fact that such priorities are no longer available in the 1970s, in a period of renewed and perhaps persistent economic decline is greatly to be deplored.

Much the same dietary recommendations are made for nursing mothers. Their normal diet needs supplementing with protective foods and *water*. The volume of water secreted in the milk is additional to the normal water losses of 2–4 pints (1–2 litres) daily, and this loss must be made good. Experiments on the value of protective foods in lactation were performed in Toronto, Canada. Supplements of milk, eggs, cheese, oranges, tomatoes, cholecalciferol and wheat germ oil were given to nursing mothers during the first 6 weeks of lactation only. The effects were still seen when the infants were 6 months old. 39% of mothers who had received the supplements were still breast-feeding, compared with 24% of those on the basal diet. Their babies were healthier and somewhat heavier. Brain growth is particularly important at this stage and is very susceptible to the baby's general health and nutritional state. If these are improved by better feeding of the nursing women then this, too, is as important as adequate nutrition during pregnancy.

Again it would be possible to determine, from the exact knowledge of the composition and volume of the milk produced, precise recommendations for the diet of the nursing mother, and to provide her with a list of these. No very great advantage will accrue from such an approach for a woman is more likely to breast feed her baby successfully if she is enjoying and digesting food she likes, than if she is made to adhere rigidly to some hypothetically correct regimen. All the weighing and measuring and the making of rules and regulations will succeed in ruining her appetite. A simple set of recommendations might be to add to the basic daily diet:

> 0.5 l of water
> 0.5 l of cow's milk
> 140 ml of fruit juice (citrus or tomato)
> *or* 150 g of fresh fruit or green vegetables
> 85 g of meat, poultry or liver
> *or* 60 g of cheese
> 1 egg

and maybe one teaspoonful of cod liver oil.

Diet and weather and climate

We all seek for different sorts of food in hot and cold weather. Hot foods and drinks are favoured in cold weather, and cold foods with iced drinks are preferred in the heat (though a special case may be made for curries and other spicy hot foods which are regularly eaten in hot climates). Pure physiology cannot explain these preferences. A whole litre of drink swallowed at 45°C can add only 34 kJ, and the same volume of ice-cold drink can remove only 155 kJ from the body. The combustion of quite a small meal liberates 2500 kJ of energy, so the amounts added by hot and cold drinks are trivial in comparison.

But why does the temperature of the drink make such a difference to one's feelings of heat, cold and comfort? The drinks alter skin temperature. We feel cold on a cold day because the blood vessels of the skin are contracted and the sense organs in the skin then register cold. A hot drink causes a reflex relaxation of the skin blood vessels, more warm blood comes to the skin and we consequently feel warm. The converse occurs when an iced drink is taken. Skin blood vessels reflexly contract and we feel cold. Curries and hot chili peppers cause a reflex onset of sweating. If the air is warm and dry the sweat evaporates and so cools the skin.

Nonetheless, there is no reason why cold foods should not be preferred in hot weather and vice versa. Our subject is *human* nutrition, and we must take the whole human being, irrational mind as well as body into consideration when planning dietaries. But one must ensure that the basic rules of physiology are followed whatever predilections weather, climate or custom may develop in us. So people should not eat less in hot weather than in cold because they do not 'feel like it'. So long as energy expenditure is the same in summer as in winter (and for many, whether it is playing tennis, gardening, hiking or other outdoor pursuits, it may be greater), then the energy content of the food must also be the same, matching the expenditure.

Within such limitations the nature of the food eaten may be altered in whatever direction appetite suggests. Hot roast beef, particularly its fat, may be repulsive in a heat wave, expecially if accompanied by potatoes roasted under the joint and Yorkshire pudding. Cold roast beef, fat and all, served with a salad and a French salad dressing may give as much energy, but is more appetising in hot weather. Amounts of fat which would be quite impossible to eat as hot beef or mutton fat are readily accepted in cream or ice-cream. Butter-fat, taken as cream on strawberries or raspberries is greatly preferred in hot weather to the same amount of butter spread on bread, or of cooking fat in sweet pastries.

Since the digestion and absorption of all foods produces a rise in heat production during the following few hours of up to 10–20% at the peak, it would clearly be best to avoid this effect coinciding with the hottest times of the day. In hot weather, the midday meal should have a low energy content, the main meals being taken early in the morning and in the evening when the temperature begins to fall. Incidentally, this effect of a meal was once thought to be due solely to the protein content of the meal. It was called the *specific dynamic action* of protein and was attributed to amino acid metabolism and the formation of the urea. Studies reported in 1972 show that even glucose will produce the same burst of heat as will protein, but with a depression in urea formation. The term specific dynamic action should be replaced with, perhaps, *thermic effect* of digestion and absorption of food. The older advice to restrict protein in hot weather is thus seen to be without foundation.

Attention should be paid to the loss of appetite in hot weather, for it may have important nutritional consequences, as well as having possible physiological causes which could be corrected.

Intense perspiration may deprive the body of salt and that makes for lassitude and lack of *joie de vivre*. Not enough water may have been drunk, so the volume of water in the tissues falls. Finally, the skin blood vessels may be widely dilated so less blood is supplied to the brain and to the gut. The reduction in salt and water content of the body will cause a fall in circulating blood volume and arterial blood pressure, accentuating the effect of increased skin blood flow. All these will result in a lack of interest in food and in a poor digestion.

The first two troubles, and in part the third can be obviated by taking plenty of salt and water. While 15 g of salt is normally more than enough in Britain, in a hot climate up to 50 g may be needed each day, and several litres of water may also be needed to replace that lost in sweat. Food should be attractive in appearance and taste, in order to stimulate the flagging appetite. Alcoholic drinks that also stimulate appetite may be taken in moderation, but not to the extent that the alcohol itself becomes an important contributor of the energy needs of the body.

Digestible and indigestible foods

Underlying many of these, and other, dietary prescriptions there is always the thought that the food must be *digestible*. This term means different things to physician, physiologist or the lay person. The latter is inclined to call *indigestible* any food that causes abdominal pain or discomfort, flatulence, or that 'repeats'. Economy minded parents might tell their children that expensive foods like shortbread biscuits are indigestible. To the scientist, it is the time taken for and the completeness of digestion and absorption that matters, and the following list of digestible and indigestible foods is largely based on these criteria.

Table 13.2 Digestible and indigestible foods.

Digestible foods	Indigestible foods
Bread, 24 hr old, dry toast, rusks, plain biscuits, porridge	New bread, scones, muffins and crumpets (hot and buttered), doughnuts
Plain sponge cakes	Fruit cakes
Butter	Meat drippings
Boiled or poached eggs	Fried eggs
White fish or lean meat, baked, boiled or grilled	Fried fish, fried meat or sausages
Chicken, turkey, guinea-fowl	Duck, goose
Floury plain boiled potatoes	Waxy boiled or chipped potatoes
Boiled young peas, beans, carrots, marrow, puréed spinach and other greens	Boiled cabbage, old carrots, turnips and swedes
Milk puddings, light steamed sponge puddings, custards, blancmanges, stewed fruit	Heavy fruit puddings, suet pudding, pastry
Fresh ripe fruit	Unripe fruit, coarse textured fruit and nuts
China tea, café au lait, cocoa	Strong tea or coffee, alcoholic drinks and aerated waters

Fats appear more frequently on the right-hand side of this table, for fat digestion is slower than that of carbohydrates or proteins, and fat slows motility of the stomach and thus delays its emptying. Cheese and bacon are not placed on the table. Many people count crisply fried bacon as digestible, despite its fat content, and many think cheese is indigestible, but 2-year-old infants can manage grated hard cheese perfectly well and some typical 'martyrs to indigestion' eat it with impunity. Even the most carefully vetted lists like the above must be considered judiciously, with reference to single persons, and not just accepted as Science-given Truth.

Economy in diet

No consideration of diets is complete without referring to their cost. It is no economy to purchase a diet cheaply if that diet does not supply sufficient energy, protein, vitamins or essential inorganic materials. On the other hand, high prices can be paid and yet a sound diet not obtained. Finally, it is no good prescribing a sound diet that is beyond the recipient's financial means. Any economical diet is one that provides the dietetic desiderata at a low price—not the lowest price, because that would probably prove too monotonous to be tolerable.

The lowest conceivable price for a diet is obtained as follows: prices for all the common foods at a given time and place are obtained. The joules, proteins and vitamins etc. obtained from each food at the cost of a penny, or the cost per megajoule or per daily requirement of protein etc. can be calculated. One then takes the amount of food that gives the minimum high biological value protein ration at the lowest cost (this will probably be cheddar cheese, though a mixture of beans and grain may be considered), calculates the joules that this would give (for cheese about 1.5 MJ) and make up the energy deficit with the cheapest energy source, probably bread and cooking margarine. This may at the same time provide enough of the B vitamins and some retinol and cholecalciferol. But this diet is ascorbic acid free, so 120 g of cabbage must be added.

Following this system, 140 g cheese, 850 g bread, 45 g margarine, 120 g cabbage perhaps form the cheapest of all possible diets. It yields 35.5 g high biological value protein and 64 g other protein, 12.5 MJ energy, 1.65 g calcium, 16 mg iron, 1.7 mg thiamine, 56 mg ascorbic acid, 0.6 mg retinol and 3.4 μg cholecalciferol. In other words, this diet approaches or actually exceeds many of the minimal requirements set by the DHSS or the American NAS. It is then a simple matter to add up its cost and obtain the smallest possible outlay that can purchase a theoretically satisfactory diet. Since food prices vary so much from place to place and time to time, there is no point in quoting figures at the time and place of writing.

It may reasonably be asked what is the point of pricing such a diet, seeing that no one could eat it day after day, or would eat it if he could. But the Royalist and Parliamentarian common soldiers of not so long ago did live, march and fight on a diet scarcely more varied than this, and in other parts of the world today many live on diets equally restricted. None the less, the calculation is of great importance for the country's social services, if not for practical dietetics, as from it social security, sickness and unemployment benefits may be determined. This is the rock-bottom price below which, or even approaching which, no subsistence allowance may go. Any alteration of this impossibly dull diet to render it more acceptable will cost more money. How much is a matter for discussion.

The present writer's father and his student worked out the minimal cost of adequate diets which they thought would be acceptable, for different ages in February 1944 in Leicester. The weekly cost of such a diet at that time for an adult male was 10s 3½d (51.5p). In 1953 it had risen to 15s 5d (77p), in 1962 to about £1 10s 6d (£1.52) and in 1971 it was well over £2. By the autumn of 1977 the whole basis of the calculations with the prices of many foods increased by different amounts in the last six years, the comparable figure must be around £4 or £5.

The principles upon which one should proceed are similar to those already described, but the range of foods must be widened and for each essential component of the diet, the cost of obtaining it from the possible sources must be calculated, and from this information the economical diet devised.

It will be found to be uneconomical to stint the protective foods. They are often omitted by the poor because of their expense. Some of them are relatively expensive, e.g. milk, eggs and fat fish, but milk at 12½p a pint is cheaper than meat as a source of protein and energy, while it contains more calcium and retinol. Margarine and butter at 11p/100 g provide energy at 3.3p/MJ, while bread (28p for a large loaf—about 830 g—in December 1977) provides it at about the same rate! But the butter and the margarine (particularly the latter) also give retinol and cholecalciferol. Eggs, regrettably, are an expensive way of providing protein, calcium, iron, vitamins or energy. Fruits and vegetables are an extremely dear way of buying energy, but are essential for ascorbic acid so cannot be omitted. Even strawberries, at the height of the season in a good year may supply ascorbic acid more cheaply than oranges, though not as cheaply as greens.

The herring once was, and the mackerel (in 1977), still is among the cheapest ways of obtaining protein, calcium, fat-soluble vitamins and iodine. The only problem here is the over-fishing which has in the last few years caused herrings to rise five-fold in price. Unless firm steps are taken to limit rigidly the number and size of mackerel caught they too will be lost as a cheap and valuable source of proteins and vitamins. At current market prices, in December 1977, cheese, ox liver and mackerel are by far the cheapest sources of animal proteins, at around 16p for 37 g protein. Then comes milk at 25p/37 g. Stewing beef, eggs and herrings cost 30–32p for 37 g and other meats and fish will be higher still.

In summary, then, it is fair to say that foods supplying animal protein, vitamins and inorganic materials are not necessarily expensive and that the usual explanation for their deficit in the British diet—their costliness—is false. The true explanation is habit, laziness and bad dietetics!

It is easiest to economise when buying energy-providing foods for two reasons. First, the protective and protein-rich foods need not exceed 30% of the energy requirements. Secondly the cost of energy-providing food varies enormously. Clearly it is easiest to economise on what forms 70% of food intake, especially when the prices range is so great. The range of cost of the day's energy supply may show a hundred-fold range whereas that for the animal protein may have only a six-fold range.

There is little point in setting out the cost per megajoule, or the cost of a day's animal protein, of the foods eaten, because of the constantly changing prices. This doesn't mean that one cannot, at any one time or place, give an estimate of the cost of a reasonable diet. The view that this could not be done, expressed by civil servants in 1932, was upset for all time by a report of the British Medical Association published in 1933. This was, in its way, perhaps as important a landmark in the history of nutrition as was the first discovery of vitamins in 1912.

Dietitians can always, given current prices and tables of food compositions, determine for any environment, the cost of ensuring an adequate diet. A general statement, true for much of Britain would be the following: 'An economical dietary must be based upon cereals and cereal products, the pulses, potatoes, milk, cheese, butter or margarine, fat fish and bacon. Meats are less economic, while eggs and lean fish are luxuries, as are any sort of convenience or pre-packed foods. Green vegetables and fruits are expensive as sources of energy, but must be included for inorganic materials and vitamins. If they can be home-grown then their quality is higher and their cost is far smaller than if they are bought at the market'.

14

Food allergy and unorthodox diets

The medical terms allergy and allergic have invaded lay speech. Tycoons are allergic to trade unions, and trade union officials to tycoons. This means that when one is mentioned to the other, they react violently.

In the same way a human body may react violently when exposed to various foreign substances, such as pollen from grasses, dust from cat, dog or horse hair, from feathers and from house-mite bodies. A person who reacts to one of these is said to be allergic to it.

Allergy is related to immunity. If foreign materials gain access to the living body they provoke defensive reactions. Often these include the production of *antibodies* which react with and neutralise the effects of the foreign material (now known as an *antigen*). Each antigen produces its own special antibody, and reactions only occur between antibodies and their 'own' antigens or closely related materials. In some cases where an antibody is fixed to a tissue, its combination with its antigen causes temporary or permanent damage to that tissue. In some, the reaction occurring in the blood provokes the severe response known as *anaphylaxis*. Mostly, however, antibodies react with their antigens smoothly and quietly so we know nothing of them. Antigens that produce any sort of untoward reaction when combining with their antibodies are called *allergens*.

A tendency to allergic reactions runs in families and so must, in part, be inheritable. Most foodstuffs can become allergens to some people, and the allergic response may be a nuisance or life-threatening. It may be difficult to track down which component of what food is in fact the allergen for a particular person. Allergens are usually, but not necessarily always, proteins, thus penicillin can become an allergen. Allergens may work in very small amounts and so traces of an antibiotic in a calf or chicken carcase may cause an allergic reaction.

In man the organs chiefly affected by food allergies are:

(1) The skin. Nettlerash or hives, urticaria, angioneurotic oedema and eczema are all thought to be allergic reactions in the skin. The exact nature of eczema is not known, but in the others the small blood vessels are affected.
(2) The respiratory tract. Hay fever is irritation of the lining of the nose, which becomes congested and causes sneezing. Asthma is contraction of bronchial muscle.
(3) The gut. Vomiting and diarrhoea are caused by irritation of mucous

membranes. Coeliac disease is a reaction to wheat protein resulting in deficient absorption of intestinal contents.
(4) The nervous system. Migraine has been ascribed to allergy.

It is by no means easy unerringly to trace what food is causing the allergy, particularly when the sufferer is taking an all-round diet containing most of the foods commonly eaten. Moreover, the offending food may cause the allergy one day and not the next. Other factors may predispose to an attack. The author's brother was, as a child, an asthmatic. Cheese and tomatoes were among the provoking substances, but they had to be accompanied by a physical or mental stress or excitement—a common cold or the onset of school holidays—before they would provoke an attack. Food allergies may only show up in the hay fever season, or during a coincident aspirin allergic response, for example.

Skin reactions, while most effective in detecting allergies to pollens, and to dusts derived from fur or feathers, are fallible when applied to foods. They give both false negative (no reaction to a food allergen) and false positive (reactions to foods not causing the allergy) results.

Three other methods are used in determining the offending foods: (1) a careful history of the food habits of the sufferer is recorded; (2) tests are made of individual suspected foods; (3) experimental diets are used.

History

If a food is an allergen and is taken only rarely, it is easy to detect it. If eating lobster is almost always followed by nettlerash, asthma or migraine, it can clearly be incriminated and avoided in future. Another example is of asthma recurring regularly on Monday, Wednesdays and Fridays in a farmer's son, who in between could be exposed to animal and threshing dusts with impunity, conditions disastrous to his cousin, also an asthmatic. The culprit was cheese, eaten for lunch on these three days. Cheese gave a positive skin test, though milk did not.

Individual food tests

If a food allergy, masked or overt, is suspected, then that food should be withheld for at least four days, and then given in a large helping. A reaction incriminates the food, but the subject should be unaware of the experiment, for he may otherwise produce an attack (a person allergic to rose pollen has been known to have an attack of asthma when he saw a bunch of artificial roses).

Experimental diets

A simple diet, giving enough energy, protein, inorganic materials and vitamins is prepared, but omitting all foods commonly known to cause allergies. If the person is free from attacks of his allergy, then after a few weeks, single foods can be added. If these do not provoke attacks, they can be incorporated into the diet and those that do can be rejected, until eventually a comprehensive list of safe and dangerous foods can be determined. The foods most frequently responsible for allergic conditions are wheat, rye, maize, eggs and milk, or any of their products. Other foods which less commonly cause problems include beef, pork, fish (especially shell fish), potatoes, the pea and bean family, oranges, tomatoes, tea, coffee, cocoa and chocolate. It must be emphasised that a sufferer from food allergy should not experiment unaided with such diets. Hearsay reports that a food, bananas, for example, caused an allergic reaction in one person are no justification for another to eliminate them from her food. People are known who collect all such 'evidence' and devise for themselves literally starvation diets as a result, with perhaps, persistence of an allergy not due to foods at all!

One condition which must be considered as an allergy is *coeliac disease*. It was not suspected as such for many years after its first medical description. It appears in childhood and the main feature is that fat absorption is defective. Other components of the diet are also poorly absorbed and coeliac disease is one of a group that lead to the nutritional deficiency state known as the *malabsorption syndrome*.

Dutch physicians discovered that the absorption defect of coeliac disease is caused by gluten, a protein found in wheat and rye. If wheat and rye, or the gluten contained in them, are removed from the foods eaten, then the disease remits. If the person unwittingly eats gluten-containing food, then the effects of the condition promptly recur. An example, from earlier days, of the effects of treatment, is that of a child whose weight had remained at 15 kg for *seven years*, yet who gained 9 kg in four months when put on a gluten free diet. It is not easy to maintain such a diet. Wheat flour is available from which the gluten has been removed. Bread and cake-making with such flour is not easy. Then many 'convenience' foods and other preparations contain wheat flour. Breakfast food cereals (e.g. Puffed Wheat, Shredded Wheat, Weetabix), bread, cakes and biscuits, pastas, suet and sponge puddings are obvious enough. Commercial ice-cream, malted milk etc., packet soups, especially thick soups, gravy browning, fish or meat pastes, bottled sauces and ketchups, salad creams, sausages and tinned meats all may and frequently do have flour in them. Unless the manufacturers disclose the composition of such foods, the unsuspecting sufferer from coeliac disease can be harmed by eating such foods.

Another condition, not an allergy, which should be mentioned here, is *lactose intolerance*. Lactose is the sugar of milk. It is normally split after absorption, within the lining cells of the intestine into its two component sugars, glucose and galactose. Almost all people are born with the enzyme necessary for splitting lactose, but may lose it completely by the time they are a year old or when they stop taking their mother's milk or any other milk. A few are born deficient in this one enzyme. In only a proportion of these, whether the deficiency is congenital or develops later in life, milk drinking leads to digestive upset. The unabsorbed lactose is attacked by bacteria and the products of this attack may lead to digestive upsets when milk is taken. This, then, is not an allergy to milk, but the consequence of drinking milk—an attack of disturbed function in the digestive system—is the same as if the person had a digestive system allergy to milk.

While on the topic of allergy, it may be well to say a few words on the unorthodox diets which turn up with such frequency. The reader may have gathered from previous remarks that the writer is allergic to such diets, which have in common one factor, their irrationality. They are not derived from scientifically gathered factual knowledge of nutrition, but depend upon some general theory, unproven or unprovable that the deviser of the diet clings to with great fervour. The body, such people say, is riddled with toxins, arising partly from the products of putrefaction in the large intestine and partly from the 'unnatural' foods eaten. These include meat (!), cereal grains raised on artificial fertiliser (nitrate, whether it comes from inorganic sodium nitrate, from bacterial decomposition of protein or urea, or from nitrogen-fixing bacteria, is all the same to a plant's protein-forming machinery—there is no way in which this can distinguish the source of the nitrogen needed for building up proteins, or the proteins can be distinguished) and refined foods such as 70% extraction flour or white sugar. These 'toxins' must be eliminated by purgation, even though there is no evidence that the large intestine absorbs anything but water and a little glucose. (It may absorb indol, a product of tryptophan, but if it did, the liver would render this substance harmless.)

It is, perhaps, correct to question both the value of inorganic fertilisers and of removing 30% of the wheat grain, but on the basis of factual knowledge obtained in agriculture or nutrition. Equally we should calmly assess the facts concerning additives to food and water, such as iodine in salt to prevent goitre, fluoride in drinking water to reduce the incidence of dental caries, or chlorine in water to prevent typhoid fever, cholera and several other infectious diseases. The first and last of these are generally accepted. Why the ferocious outbreaks of emotion over fluoride? They have no basis in reason.

On the other hand, the unorthodox may seize upon a new discovery, such as vitamins, trace materials or fibre, and then misapply it in his search for a new dietary regimen. If there is some 'magical' element, or one of return to 'the good old days', then he is keen to follow it. Thus cider vinegar is preferred to malt vinegar, brown sugar to white, honey to any form of sugar and black treacle to golden syrup. Foreign and unusual foods are chosen, like yoghourt from eastern Europe or Maté tea from South America (ordinary milk and tea from India are too common!). Often one can detect a trace of sadism and masochism in the fervour with which the unorthodox pursue their regimes, but always the prescribers *know the truth*. They are, in fact, releasing the irrational side of their make-up. This may even be of value to them, being an escape from the burden of rationality. The dietitian must expect that people will be more irrational over food, say, than over cars or clothes, for feeding is the earliest activity over which the baby gets emotional.

All this is not to say that unorthodox diets may not do some people good. Migraine sufferers have benefited, and it is clear that organic fertilisers may be better for farm land than inorganic, while wholewheat bread and black treacle are known to be better than white bread and white sugar on sound nutritional evidence. Whatever diet one selects, it must contain adequate protein, energy, vitamins and inorganic materials. It is no use concentrating on one of these and neglecting the rest. A diet of orange juice, lettuce and raw cabbage will give retinol and ascorbic acid, and perhaps calcium and iron, but by no means enough protein or energy.

Here is an unorthodox diet claimed to be useful in lowering arterial blood pressure and body weight and in treating 'rheumatism'.

Early morning
'Blood cleansing drink', i.e. an infusion of vegetable purgatives
Breakfast
Dried fruits, previously soaked for 48 hours. Fresh fruits *ad libitum*
Mid-morning
Maté tea or dandelion coffee
Lunch
56 g or more cheese, raw vegetable salad, baked potato, yoghourt and brown sugar, wholemeal bread and butter
Mid-afternoon
Maté or green tea
Evening meal
Cheese or egg dish, baked potato, wholemeal bread and butter

At various meals vitamin concentrates were given (perhaps unnecessarily) and twice a day a drink made from expressed and centrifuged vegetable and fruit cell fluids.

The sceptical dietitian can find little wrong with this diet, though it is in many ways irrational. It provides enough energy, protein, vitamins and inorganic materials. Maybe the light breakfast and the absence of meat will upset some, and others might find that deprivation of tea would cause them trouble. The present writer has never experienced such a diet, but his father says it caused a fall in blood pressure and weight (both beneficial), but also produced mental depression. It may well affect other people in different ways.

15
Food hygiene

In a practical book on human nutrition it is essential to make some mention of food hygiene. The dietitian is seen to encourage the consumption of, say, watercress, milk, or even of ice-cream. Opposition to watercress may come from the fear of typhoid fever, transmitted by untreated human sewage entering our rivers, though this is most unlikely now in Britain. Milk undoubtedly transmits typhoid fever, tuberculosis and undulant fever. In 1936 in Bournemouth milk transmission caused a typhoid epidemic of 178 cases with 51 deaths, while in 1946 in Aberystwyth a single ice-cream vendor spread typhoid to many people. Apart from the distress to the sufferers, which cannot be measured, there was a considerable economic loss in both cases due to cancelled holidays etc.

The subject of food hygiene, then, has a twofold aspect, community and personal or domestic. Much of the production, storage and distribution of food is done by large-scale government-controlled concerns, as is that of drinking water. Thus the authorities (national or local governmental) must inspect slaughterhouses, food factories, dairies and bakeries. They are also responsible for water supplies and the disposal of sewage and domestic refuse. In all these, the private citizen has no control, though well-informed tax and ratepayers can maintain a high standard from official inspectors. The same authorities have acted with commendable speed and efficiency in tracking down the cause of food-borne epidemics, though if the Ministries had earlier taken standards of production into their purview, and if there was always an adequate follow up of every person suffering from diseases that may be food-borne, then the epidemics might have been prevented. Since so much of our food already undergoes so many preparative processes before it reaches the home, and since this centralisation will continue to increase, the national control of food hygiene must also increase. It is the government's business to deal directly, or indirectly through adequately financed local authorities, with the water supply, with milk and dairy produce, with meat, poultry and egg production, with the public fruit and vegetable markets and to see that in all high standards of health and cleanliness are maintained. Each citizen has his or her share, also, of reponsibility, of knowing the risks run, of understanding, accepting and obeying such simple rules as hand-washing and restricting access of dogs to foodshops, and in keeping the responsible authorities up to the mark.

Diseases transmitted by foods

Foods act as passive vectors of many infectious diseases, while in other cases the infective organism actively grows in the food before it is eaten, or liberates into the food poisonous products of its metabolism. Members of most classes of parasitic and infective organism may enter the human body by way of food. Among virus infections, poliomyelitis and coxsackie viruses are primarily gastroenteric infections and they may be carried on foods. While typhoid fever and tuberculosis are the best-known bacterial diseases that may infect man by foods, there are many others. Amoebic dysentery is an important protozoal disease in tropical countries, for the infective organism readily gains access to food. In all parts of the world tapeworms may be transmitted in beef, pork or fish, and pork also conveys trichiniasis to man. Many bacteria, on gaining access to and living in prepared foods, produce heat-stable toxic products which survive death of the bacteria themselves. Commonest among these are various *Salmonella* species, clostridia (which thrive best in an oxygen-free environment), and organisms, such as staphylococci and streptococci which are common inhabitants of the human skin and throat (where they may cause boils etc. and sore throats). *Clostridium botulinum* produces a very powerful neuromuscular poison, but the rest produce toxins that are intensely irritant to the stomach and intestines. These toxins cause the typical 'food-poisoning' attack, an acute onset of vomiting and diarrhoea which usually lasts 24–48 hours only. While not usually serious, such attacks may be fatal and are always unpleasant. Many other food-borne diseases may cause the same symptoms but in these the onset is usually more gradual and the disturbances of gastrointestinal tract function more persistent. The distinction between *infections*, such as typhoid fever and the dysenteries (in which it is bacteria living in the gut's contents and walls that cause the trouble), and the *food poisonings* (in which it is the products of dead bacteria that are toxic), must be remembered. Heat treatment of infected food will kill the bacteria, but will not destroy the toxins that may have already formed. Some bacteria may cause both types of illness. Thus *Salmonella typhi* which causes typhoid fever can produce powerful exotoxins if it is allowed to grow in food, as also can the *Streptococcus* that causes sore throats and scarlet fever. Both organisms have produced 'food-poisoning' attacks, and both may gain access, still alive, to the body in infected solid foods, milk or water, causing typhoid or scarlet fevers.

Some of the infecting organisms, the clostridia for example, are widely distributed in the soil, manures and intestines of many animals, including man. Staphylococci and streptococci inhabit many a healthy person's skin, nose and throat, while after an attack of typhoid fever, the bacterium may live on for many years, unsuspected, in kidneys or the gall bladder, being excreted therefrom in urine or faeces respectively. Other *Salmonella* species which cause food-poisoning attacks live similarly in rodents, cockroaches etc. Tuberculosis and undulant fever deserve special mention. The causative organism of the former, *Mycobacterium tuberculosis*, has adapted to live in different animal species, including the cow. Infected cows may excrete living bacteria in their milk, and bovine tuberculosis in man is caused by drinking this infected milk. It usually runs a different course from tuberculosis caused by the human strain of the organism. A child with tuberculosis glands of the neck is probably suffering from a milk-borne, bovine infection, but one with 'a spot on his lung' has probably contracted human tuberculosis, by inhaling living mycobacteria, coughed out by another sufferer from the disease. Undulant fever is a generalised chronic febrile illness caused by infection with strains of *Brucella* (hence the alternative name, brucellosis). One strain commonly infects cows, from which it is transmitted, like tuberculosis, in the milk. In cows it causes septic abortions, so this strain of *Brucella* is called *Br. abortus*. Goats are the natural host of another strain of *Brucella* which, since it was first isolated in Malta, is known as *Br. melitensis*. The Maltese variety of undulant fever is a more severe disease than that caused by *Br. abortus*, so it was many years after the cause of the Maltese disease was isolated that attention was turned to the bovine variety of undulant fever.

Many of the multicelled (metazoal) parasites that enter the human body in food undergo complicated life-cycles involving two species of host animals. Adult worms commonly live in the gut and their eggs are shed in the faeces. An intermediate stage may exist, in which the immature organism lies dormant in cysts scattered throughout the body, including the muscles and liver. For details of the fascinating life-cycles of some of these creatures, a zoology text should be studied. Adult tapeworms in our guts are more a nuisance than harmful, except the rare *Diphyllobothrium latum*, which is so avid for cobalamin that those infected by it develop anaemia. A roundworm, *Ascaris lumbricoides* (that is, it looks like an earthworm), may also cause anaemia due to its diet of the host's blood. Its eggs are shed into the faeces, whence they may gain access to food and so pass on the infestation to a new host.

Now that the nature of the food-borne diseases and their causative organisms have been described, the importance of food hygiene should be apparent. The means of preventing these diseases, both in the community at large, and in the single household will now be described.

Communal control of food hygiene

People who have survived an attack of typhoid fever may become, as already mentioned, life-long carriers, excreting living *S. typhi* in their urine or faeces. From inadequately treated sewage the organisms may enter water supplies and thus infect other people. The organisms may also get onto the carrier's hands and thence to foods if the carrier is working at any stage in the food-processing or distribution industries. It is thus of great importance to the public health authority to ensure that carriers are not present in food factories, abattoirs, shops or restaurants, and that all such workers at these places are very careful in all matters of personal hygiene. The employers should ensure that hand-washing facilities are at least as good as in their own homes and that their workers wash after attending to their bodily needs.

People with sore hands, faces or throats, or suffering from boils and similar skin infections should not be allowed to prepare food.

Various foods can become infected from the surroundings in which they grow. Thus watercress, if the beds are supplied with infected water, may convey the infection to man. Oysters and other molluscs actively filter out micro-organisms from the surrounding water for their own food. Again, if the water is infected, the organism is filtered out by the shellfish and subsequently passed to man when he eats the oyster. Another example of passive carriage of an infectious organism is the typhoid fever epidemic of 1964, centred upon Aberdeen. It is practically certain that the food which started this epidemic was a single ten-pound tin of corned beef. This tin had been sealed and heat sterilised in the usual way. How then did its contents become contaminated with *S. typhi*? The tin came from a country where typhoid fever is widespread, and the tins were cooled after sterilisation in water which had not been treated with chlorine to kill any living micro-organisms. It is assumed that the incriminated tin had some small aperture through which the *S. typhi* in the river water could enter and infect the contents. Not only was this block of corned beef infected, but the infection spread to the knives used in cutting it and thus to other cold cooked meats sold in the same shop. Finally, it was known that the cooling water was unchlorinated, but nothing had been done about this by the manufacturer or the health authorities in the country concerned.

The problems of infected milk have been tackled in two ways. The first is by heat treatment, *pasteurisation* of the milk, which destroys the disease-causing micro-organisms. When pasteurisation was applied to 50% of London's milk there were still 136 deaths from bovine tuberculosis per year per million inhabitants, but when the process was virtually universal the death rate fell to 4. Similar falls have been seen in other areas. The second approach has been to eradicate the diseases tuberculosis and contagious abortion from the dairy herds, and to keep them disease-free. For bovine tuberculosis the eradication programme is virtually complete in Britain (though some suspect that badgers may be re-infecting dairy herds), but progress has been slower with *Br. abortus* infection, perhaps because human brucellosis is not so severe as tuberculosis once was.

Foods may become contaminated by any of the animals that commonly hang around human habitations. Among these are mice and rats, cockroaches, flies and dogs. There is no place for any of these where foods are being prepared for human consumption. The rodents certainly, and cockroaches probably convey to food various *Salmonella* species which cause food-poisoning attacks. Flies, feeding alternately on faeces and food, will convey micro-organisms from one to the other. Dogs are hosts for the adult stage of the tapeworm *Taenia echinococcus*, and man can be a host for its intermediate stage if eggs gain access from the dogs' faeces to human food. It is for this reason that food retailers in Britain discourage the access of dogs, whether household pets or otherwise, to their premises.

All these matters, detection of carriers, effective treatment of sewage and drinking water, the elimination of rodents, dogs and insects, and the ensuring of high standards of personal cleanliness in all places where foods are processed or distributed, are the responsibility of the public health authorities, and are aimed at ensuring that the foods brought into our homes, or eaten at restaurants are both wholesome and safe for us to eat.

Food hygiene in the home

This is an extension of the same principles that apply in the previous section. Carriers of food-poisoning micro-organisms may infect their own or their families' food. Waste and infection must be avoided by excluding moulds, putrefying and souring bacteria, flies, cockroaches, mice and rats from the food. Failure to use crusts of bread, or to clear out stale bread-crumbs from the bread-bin, leads to mould growing over whole loaves. Lazy scattering or neglect of scraps of food encourages unwanted animal life, with the resultant waste of more food becoming fouled by such animals. Food may similarly be spoiled by house flies, including the bluebottle and blowfly. These lay their eggs on exposed meat or bacon, whence the grubs hatch out and grow rapidly in warm weather, spoiling the meat. The adult flies, as already seen, can at the same time as laying their eggs, contaminate the food with unwanted bacteria. If the British fly and mosquito were even more prevalent, then perhaps we would learn from North America and protect our houses with fly-proof screens over doors and windows.

Refrigerators can do a great deal towards preventing food wastage in the home. Not only do they keep food cold, and so greatly reduce the rate of bacterial growth, but since they have to be air-tight to work properly, they are also fly-proof, and proof against cockroaches, mice and rats. As an example of the value of the domestic refrigerator, in the USA the present writer bought pasteurised milk in waxed cartons at a local supermarket and stored it in his refrigerator where it remained wholesome for as much as a week.

Where there is no refrigerator the ordinary housewife must use her intelligence to keep food sweet. Meats, especially when raw, are most likely to be spoilt and made dangerous by bacterial growth. If cooking must be delayed, the meat should be suspended in air, so its surface can become dry, which reduces bacterial growth. On bringing food from room to cooking temperature, this should be done as rapidly as possible, to minimise the time during which the meat is at a temperature suitable for rapid bacterial growth. Casserole-type dishes with close fitting lids are useful, although such kitchen utensils do not fulfil the conditions of Spallanzani's and Pasteur's original experiments on putrefaction of cooked meats and vege-tables, which showed that this only began if air obtained free access to the food after cooking. This writer has found that a saucepan containing stew may keep for some days, even at British summer temperature, if the lid is not disturbed once the stew has boiled for 5 minutes. This rule can be generally applied to any 'left overs'. If they can be put, in a covered container, into the larder undisturbed after being thoroughly heated through, they will keep fresh for some days, even without the use of a refrigerator.

While the domestic refrigerator is becoming common in Britain nowadays, the deep-freeze cabinet is adding a new dimension to domestic economy, and to food hygiene matters. Many foods are now bought frozen and wrapped in bacteria and fly-proof packs that used to be bought from open shops and markets. These can be stored for days or weeks in the home refrigerator or freezer unit and used as required. In some cases a loss of quality may occur with injudicious thawing and re-freezing, but common sense can obviate any danger. The deep-freeze can also be used for storing left-overs, which will be as wholesome when re-thawed as they were when initially frozen. One must remember always that living bacteria are not necessarily destroyed by freezing, and that once a thawed article of food reaches a high enough temperature, then bacterial growth will recommence. Thawed foods must be cooked, or re-cooked as soon as is practicable.

The remaining most important aspect of kitchen hygiene is to have plenty of hot running water and soap or detergent for the cleaning of food utensils. Soap and detergents are moderately efficient antiseptics, though they do not kill all types of bacteria and are ineffective against bacterial spores (e.g. the clostridia). It is perhaps best to rinse the utensils in fresh hot water after washing in soap or detergent solution, and leave them to dry in the air. Drying cloths may harbour bacteria that have become resistant to soaps etc. and re-contaminate the utensils with these micro-organisms.

Finally, the embargo on the domestic dog in retail food shops should be extended to the kitchen at home, particularly in areas where *Taenia echinococcus* is common. Household pets should always have their own utensils which are kept separate at all times from those used by the human inhabitants, and their food waste must be removed just as is our own, to prevent the encouragement of other pests.

In this chapter, the possibilities of transmitting disease by food has been emphasised—some may say too much emphasised. It is certainly true that the stress laid in the past on the dirtiness of milk (bacteriologically speaking) has prejudiced people against milk as a food, and the campaign for clean milk has worked against the increase of milk consumption. There is a danger in giving the public an exaggerated fear of bacteria, but the real danger must be faced. People should understand the ubiquity, the services and the disservices of bacteria and how to take advantage of the one and avoid the other. Much of the control of the harmful effects is in the hands of the public authorities, but this must be backed up by an educated public opinion. It may reasonably be said, however, that in Great Britain, due to the efforts of the authorities, there is now little disease traceable to the contamination of food with bacteria or other parasites, though it must be confessed that when these enemies to health and life get under our guard the results can be devastating. Thus in the olden days, everyone was exposed in infancy or childhood to such diseases as bovine tuberculosis, typhoid fever, poliomyelitis, 'summer diarrhoeas' of many types. A few died but the majority recovered with no ill effects, and a life-long immunity. The price of saving all from childhood infection and a few from death is eternal vigilance on the part of us all.

After this chapter had been completed in December 1977, a report was published on food-poisoning attacks in the last few years which rose from 140 in 1972 to 260 in 1975 and to nearly 500 in 1976. While sporadic and individual household attacks were not changing in frequency, 1976 was thus the fourth successive year to show an increase in attacks affecting several households simultaneously, that is, due to infection at a catering or food manufacturing establishment. Between 6000 and 10 000 people were affected. *Salmonella* species were by far the commonest organism causing the attacks, and the vehicles were meats, poultry and stocks or sauces prepared from meat. The bacteria may be present in the animals before slaughtering, and poor standards of hygiene in those handling the foods or inadequate thawing and cooking of frozen material may be contributory factors in causing this increase. The report serves to underline the comments already made in this chapter about personal care among food handlers, but also raises the problem of infection of living animals prior to slaughter. This perhaps becomes a matter of applying knowledge of human infectious diseases to animal husbandry. It is not enough to feed chickens and calves with antibiotics. The bacteria readily become immune to these, and the traces that get into human food may do further harm. Nothing promotes bacterial resistance to antibiotics as well as repeated exposure to small amounts of these materials. Fundamental alterations in present methods of rearing food-animals may have to be adopted, which will affect yet again our eating habits.

16
Cooking, processing and storage of food in relation to nutritional value

Many foods in their natural state cannot be digested by man, e.g. cereals, pulses, potatoes, and so must be 'processed' before eating. A home 'process' is that of cooking, which has been practised from before the dawn of recorded history. Possibly cooking was first applied to cereals, though some think that prehistoric man learnt the value of cooking his preferred food, meat.

Any book on human nutrition must, then, consider the advantages and disadvantages of cooking and other methods of food processing. A syllogistic argument is often advanced. Animals don't cook foods. Man is an animal. Therefore man should not cook foods. This has been, and is, proposed seriously. What can one say against such an *a priori* argument?

One must look at the factual evidence. Cooking (and many other processes) increases the palatability, digestibility, the keeping qualities and the safety of foods. Are these advantages accompanied by a loss in any food value? The true factual answer is: sometimes. It is a case of compromise, but we will anticipate the details and say that the best compromise is nearer to having all foods cooked than all raw.

Chemical changes induced by cooking

Proteins

Proteins are irreversibly altered or *denatured* by the heat of boiling water. Many, previously in solution in water, form a coagulum or gel at this temperature, binding the water into a 'water in protein' form of colloid state. Insoluble collagen, the chief protein of connective tissue is converted to soluble gelatin at 100°C which only forms a gel with water when cooled. Dry heat, as in roasting, baking or frying, when the temperature exceeds 100°C, takes some of the protein near to its charring point, developing highly flavoured substances and probably reducing its value as body-building material. There is both gain and loss in cooking proteins. The conversion of collagen to gelatin renders meats far more friable, so teeth can break them up and the proteolytic enzymes can penetrate the meat more effectively. Gelatin itself is more readily attacked by these enzymes than the original collagen. Boiled egg albumin loses its affinity for the vitamin biotin. Boiled caseinogen forms smaller, more digestible curds in the stomach than does raw caseinogen. In some cases the biological value of individual proteins is raised and in others it is lowered by cooking. The gain of highly flavoured and appetising roast meat has to be offset by a fall in its biological value. While in theory we cannot fully evaluate the balance between good and evil, since we do not have all the evidence, in practice, the possible disadvantages of cooking proteins cannot be great, or the human race would not have survived so many thousands of years of cooking proteins!

Fats

No very obvious changes take place unless the heat be dry and fierce as in rapid shallow frying, in grilling or roasting. Peroxides and irritant substances such as acrolein may be formed from some polyunsaturated fatty acids. These may cause indigestion. One anecdote even speaks of peptic ulcers being cured by a change from shallow to deep frying!

Starches

Dry heating turns raw starch into dextrins which are much more water-soluble and readily attacked by amylases. Boiling converts the raw starch of potatoes or wheat flour into soluble starch, which again can be attacked by digestive amylases. Thus both forms of cooking render starch more digestible.

Sugars

Both wet and dry heating have effects on the disaccharides, sucrose, maltose and lactose. Only the former need concern us here. Wet heat, particularly in the presence of fruit acid, hydrolyses one molecule of sucrose into one each of glucose and fructose. It is doubtful if these are more digestible or absorbable than sucrose, though the process is of importance in jam making, for the mixture of the two monosaccharides has twice the osmotic effect of the parent sucrose and so restricts the growth of moulds etc.

Cellulose

This indigestible carbohydrate is found in plant cell walls. Cooking disrupts these and so the contents of plant cells, which cannot be attacked by digestive enzymes when the plant materials are eaten raw, become available after cooking. There is no doubt that cooked carrots are more digestible than raw carrots, boiled greens than raw cabbage. Raw greens produce flatulence and indigestion in some, though others can eat them with no ill effects.

So with all carbohydrate materials the balance is clearly in favour of cooking, especially in foods containing starch and unbroken cell walls.

Vitamins

Ascorbic acid is the only vitamin that is readily destroyed by cooking. More is lost by being dissolved into the cooking water and so poured down the sink. Careful, minimal cooking can however preserve sufficient ascorbic acid to make it unnecessary to insist on raw vegetables being part of the daily diet. While pressure cooking elevates the temperature still further, the time of cooking is reduced and while boiled potatoes may lose half their ascorbic acid, in a pressure cooker they may only lose one fifth of the original content. Some thiamine and folic acid may be destroyed by cooking. Thiamine may also be extensively lost into the water used in boiling rice if excess water is used.

Inorganic materials

Wet cooking may leach out some magnesium and potassium from foods, but hardly affects calcium or iron or any of the other materials. It is thus nonsense to talk of the 'valuable mineral salts' being lost in cooking processes.

The other advantages of cooking

In most cases, cooked food is more palatable than the same food when raw, though one must remember that our preferences in this may be conditioned and not inborn. As already mentioned, most meats become tender on cooking and this is a great advantage. Moreover, cooking produces new flavours in the major foodstuffs, providing also the advantage of variety in flavours.

Similarly, cooking enhances digestibility of meats, pulse and grain seeds and of vegetables. This refers correctly to attack of constituent components of the food by the digestive enzymes in a test tube. It is assumed that digestibility is also enhanced in the gut, wherein the greater pleasure derived from eating the well-flavoured cooked foods will lead to a greater production of the digestive enzymes.

The keeping quality of foods is greatly enhanced by cooking which not only kills adventitious bacteria which may spoil the food in any one of several different ways, but also inactivates the enzymes within the cells of the food which themselves might render it inedible. Cooked food that is then sealed off from the environment and its micro-organisms will keep indefinitely. Tins of meat, sealed over 100 years ago, were still edible when opened. Even though exposed to air, a joint of meat will keep for several days after roasting, especially if it is kept dry and free from flies and mice.

Cooking also makes foods safer. It destroys bacteria and parasitic worms or their eggs, although some exotoxins produced by bacteria are heat stable (e.g. those formed by *Salmonella* species). *C. botulinum* toxin is destroyed by cooking.

On the other side of the argument, cooking can and does become a time and energy consuming obsessional activity—witness the endless supply of cookery books and of recipes in the weekly and monthly women's magazines. Furthermore, cooking *can* be used to hide defects in food. Nothing but the best can be served raw, but unpleasant flavours and worse can be obscured by cooking, especially with the addition of highly flavoured spices etc. Cooking does reduce the ascorbic acid content of all vegetables. Thus brussels sprouts contain 100 mg/100 g when purchased, but only 30 mg/100 g at the best when cooked. Even so this amount, in a normal serving, is more than enough to maintain adequate ascorbic acid levels in a healthy person. Raw food diets have been used in Britain for treating diseases and dramatic cures, even of tuberculosis, have been claimed. Success is more readily achieved with osteoarthrosis (formerly osteo-arthritis), but since raw-food diets are low in sodium chloride and reduce weight, it is more probably these factors that improve the patients' condition rather than the large amount of ascorbic acid or some as yet unknown factor destroyed by cooking. It may well be that the healthy surroundings, enthusiasm and optimism played as much part in the results claimed as any dietary factor.

In conclusion, then, the objective or scientifically minded dietitian is forced to accept that the balance of evidence is definitely in favour of cooking foods, but that to obviate one of its disadvantages, the destruction of ascorbic acid, some raw or very lightly cooked green salad is desirable each day, or some fresh citrus fruit, which is now available all the year around. Even here we do not wish to become obsessional. Provided one does not break a bone or undergo major surgery, one can remain healthy for some months on the daily intake of about 10 mg ascorbic acid that can easily be obtained from home-cooked potatoes and greens.

Institutional cooking

It is particularly difficult in all whole-time institutions to obtain a wholly satisfactory and satisfying dietary. While the food may be nutritionally adequate, it is frequently unappetising. The defects are mainly the result of mass-production as opposed to craftsman techniques, but have a distinct bearing on dietetics.

Montony

A catering institution has a better chance of serving well-cooked meat than the home. Joints may be larger, and the apparatus much better. But this perfection of cooking in the best of hotels may become monotonous, and the variations from the normal produced in domestic cookery add the spice of variety to the foods. In large-scale cookery, for example, the amounts of seasoning are weighed and thus bear an exact and un-varying ratio to the other ingredients. A dish made from the same recipe is always the same and soon becomes monotonous. In the home there are shakes of the pepper pot, pinches of salt, or 'as much as ought to be enough' of herbs or other flavouring. A dish never comes out exactly the same no matter how often it is repeated.

'The need to keep things hot'

It must be realised that 'dishing up' in a big establishment takes much longer than in the home—perhaps not in proportion to the amounts served, but in actual time. That results, for example in the potatoes and the vegetables having to be kept hot for a longer time than in the home. In a restaurant or works canteen, serving lunches between 12 noon and 2 p.m., it is quite possible that the potatoes or brussels sprouts served at 1.30 p.m.

were actually dished up at 11.45 a.m. and had been kept hot ever since. Quite apart from the decline in palatability during that time, the ascorbic acid content will have declined to negligible amounts.

Labour saving in preparation

Time is money in any institution, and labour time is extremely costly nowadays. In a single household, a half hour spent in shelling peas for the family (while sitting and enjoying the garden) is time well spent. It would be quite impossible to do the same thing in a hotel, hospital or factory kitchen. The peas are bought ready shelled and either canned or frozen. A diner will notice that such peas are all of the same size, and if he has an eye for colour, that this suggests an added dye. The simple fact is that you cannot get 'garden peas' in any institution. The commercial grower will not pick peas that are young and only partly grown. The canner and freezer sieves the peas so that each container is filled with peas of exactly the same size. The delightful variety of size and texture of home-picked peas is not available to the institutional caterer, but he can serve peas of reliable quality on any day of the year.

Institutions and individuals

Earlier in this book it has been indicated that individuals count in dietetics and that it is no use treating everyone as if he were an 'average person'. The 'reasonable man on the Clapham omnibus' is as much a nutritional as he is a legal fiction. This becomes most apparent when considering institutional feeding. The writer has lived for long periods in a boarding school and a residential club and has sampled many different institutions' midday meals and restaurant catering. Nothing makes the members of these institutions more cantankerous than the food they provide. Thus my own most unpleasant memory of a stay in one of the country's foremost teaching hospitals concerns the food provided there—though I was and am still quite unable to state objectively what was wrong with it! Probably part of the basis for the unfavourable psychological reactions is the inevitable monotony of institutional food. This is perhaps partly due to lack of knowledge and imagination on the part of the caterer, and partly due to the standardisation forced by the need to save money. Since all health and fitness have a sound dietary as their foundation, it is clear that all institutions need better dietetic supervision than the home. It is, moreover, as well that any dietitian employed in an institution should from time to time live as one of the inmates, and learn what really goes on there, in dining-hall or common-room, as well as in the kitchen, store-room or office

Other modes of preserving and processing food

Cooking of foods does help to preserve them for short periods of time, but there has always been a need to keep foods for long enough in most of the world to enable people to survive seasonal or longer changes in food supply.

The Nile Valley, one of the early sites of urban civilisation, has always depended on the annual inundation due to heavy seasonal rainfall in Ethiopia, and longer term changes in its food production were experienced in the time of Joseph. In the present age, with distribution of food on a world-wide basis, seasonal or other changes in one region need not be so important as formerly. Nonetheless, it is still necessary to consider how storage methods might affect nutritional quality.

Drying

Drying is the oldest and simplest method. Bacteria grow much less readily, if at all, in dried materials than in moist. Drying concentrates any water-soluble substances, such as sugars, which in concentrated solution exert such an osmotic effect as to prevent the growth of moulds and yeasts. Nature, indeed, has anticipated man in this. Seeds are dried embryonic plants, with a varying amount of dried food material attached. Seeds will survive ('keep') over periods of drought or cold, even for several years. The best keeping foods are thus seeds, grain or pulses which, except in a damp climate or growing season, need no extra drying to make them last.

Meats have been dried, either in strips or as mince, in many countries, according to methods learned long ago. In a modern process, a side of beef weighing 68 kg and occupying 1.78 m^3 of space can be converted into a 20 kg block, occupying 0.28 m^3. It would be dried at 80°C, after cooking and mincing, until it contained 7.5% water. It would then be packed, in nitrogen, in airtight containers and would keep for a year. The nutritional value would be unharmed by this process, except for the partial loss of thiamine. Dried fish, fruit and vegetables have similarly existed from ancient times, and modern industrial processes have been developed, as outlined above for meat. The dried fruit and vegetables have probably little or no ascorbic acid, so their widespread use instead of fresh products in times of scarcity may lead to outbreaks of scurvy.

Drying of surplus milk has become a widespread practice. Do what they will, farmers cannot persuade cows in a temperate climate to produce the same amount of milk each day throughout the seasonal changes of the year. Cheese making (to be considered later) is one way of managing the problem. Another is to dry the milk (with its fat or after skimming) and store the powder for distribution as and where it is needed. Milk is dried either on steam-heated rollers, or by spraying into a heated chamber. In both methods some thiamine is lost and the biological value of the proteins is reduced somewhat. When reconstituted with water it does not taste like fresh milk, but, like boiled milk, it is better digested by infants than is fresh milk.

To simple drying, especially of vegetables, other techniques may be added that will preserve some of the labile vitamins, ascorbic acid and thiamine. The first is *blanching*. This is simply a brief period of cooking, sufficient merely to inactivate destructive enzymes. It may then be followed by rapid drying (preferably free from oxygen) and the product contains a reasonable proportion of its original vitamin content. A second method is *freeze drying*. In this the foodstuff is first frozen (about which much more later) and then prolonged drying, while frozen, will remove the water directly from the ice in the material—a process known to chemists as *sublimation*, in which solid is converted to gas without passing through a liquid phase. Once the product is water-free it can be packed and stored at room temperature indefinitely. It is a costly process, but as storage is so easy and cheap it may prove eventually to be a favourable method economically.

Smoking   DOPE RULES

Many meats and fish can have their keeping quality and flavour enhanced if the drying process is accompanied by exposure to smoke from hardwood. Herring, haddock, ham, bacon and many sausages are preserved by drying with smoke. It is thought that formaldehyde, a product of smoking combustion of wood, which is antiseptic, may enhance the keeping of smoked products.

Salting

Salting has also been used from prehistoric time, sometimes along with drying, to preserve foods. Dry salt (frequently containing potassium nitrate along with the sodium chloride) may be rubbed into meat, which is then dried, or the meat may be packed into containers filled with strong salt solution. In either case the bacteria cannot grow in the salty medium. Dry salting is usually followed by drying or smoking as additional preservative techniques. Both wet and dry salting are usually applied to meat and fish, but were also, before freezing became widespread, applied to vegetable preservation.

Cold

After drying in various forms, the use of low temperatures is a most widely used method of preserving foods. A reduction of temperature reduces the rates of chemical reactions on which living processes depend, and there are few enzyme-promoted reactions or whole living organisms that proceed or grow at significant rates when the temperature is reduced to 0°C. Lower temperatures are even more effective, but the development of ice crystals in the foods so cooled spoils their quality in some cases. Foods must be separated into those that can be *deep frozen*, with ice formation, and those that can only be *chilled*, to around 0°C. The techniques of mechanical refrigeration are the same in both cases, but chilling may also be achieved, by the fuel-conscious, with the use of natural ice, cut from lakes in the winter and stored in insulated ice houses to last through the summer. Ice is also widely used where mechanical refrigeration is not practicable, e.g. on the fishmonger's slab, to keep his wares fresh and fit to sell.

Cooling techniques inevitably vary with the food to be preserved. Sides of lamb can be frozen solid, but beef cannot, for the inevitably slow rate of cooling of the large mass allows large ice crystals to develop within the tissue. These cause disruption of the cells and excessive fluid loss and alteration of texture when the meat is subsequently thawed. Individual slices of beef-steak can, however, be deep-frozen sufficiently quickly to prevent large ice-crystals from forming. The storage of chilled beef carcases presents a real technical problem as the European common market has found in the 1970s, but both chilling and deep-freezing has enabled meat to be shipped around the world in a manner that would have been quite impossible before cooling methods were developed.

Smaller objects than carcases of meat are best frozen rapidly by exposure either to a saturated salt solution at −20°C or to liquid nitrogen at −187°C. Fish, fruit and many vegetables are frozen by these techniques and a whole new industry has developed since the 1950s in Britain concerned with the preparation, distribution and domestic storage of deep-frozen foodstuffs. Wholly new foods, the fish finger, for example, have been developed. Many other foods with only a limited cropping season have become available in a state only marginally less satisfactory than the freshly collected, throughout the year. The domestic deep-freeze unit has allowed the individual household to prepare its own foods for storage. Many summer fruits need only to be placed in sealed, water-vapour impermeable containers before being frozen. Others must be cooked first (apples, for example) since they spoil, due to enzyme action, on thawing. Vegetables for the same reason, should be blanched and rapidly cooled before being frozen. Fish should be gutted and filleted if necessary, then washed and frozen quickly.

Partly prepared foods, or foods cooked and ready for eating can also be deep-frozen. Frozen yeast doughs, bread, fruit cakes and fruit tarts or pies, for example—even complete cream slices—can be frozen, either commercially or in the home freezer, and then brought out and thawed, further cooked or eaten as occasion demands.

The advent of these methods, though they may be expensive in equipment and running fuel costs, have resulted in a greatly increased potential for a more varied, and therefore improved, dietary in countries sufficiently wealthy to allow every village store to have its deep-freeze cabinets. The author's own experience when, early in the 1960s, he purchased a domestic freezer, was that his family lived better, on a more varied diet for the same cost than formerly, also that freezing surplus vegetable garden produce gave a better and more reliable product than the wet-salting method that he had used for some years previously.

Sterilisation and canning or bottling

If any fresh food is heated to 100°C this will destroy all living bacteria (some bacterial spores will survive at up to 125°C and re-heating to 100°C at successive intervals of time is needed to deal with them). If, after this sterilising process, the food is then sealed with a leak-proof container it will keep indefinitely. Home bottling of fruit or vegetables has long been accepted as a domestic industry, and commercial canning has been widespread for over 100 years. Some foods, such as sardines or kidney beans are virtually only known in Britain in their popular canned varieties and it has been said in peach-growing areas that 'we eat what we can, and can what we can't'. But the canned peach is a very different article from the fresh one and, since a concentrated syrup is always added to canned fruit, this has a much higher energy content than the fresh fruit. But the quotation illustrates once again the importance of the preserving technique. Surpluses are saved for a time when climate prevents fresh goods being available. The change in availability must be set against any change in quality.

Pasteurisation is a technique of partial sterilisation that has been widely applied to milk, though it may be applied to other liquids (Pasteur originally devised the technique as an aid to more reliable fermentation of grape juice). The food is raised to a temperature and held there for a time sufficient to kill unwanted micro-organisms. A temperature of 62°C, held for 30 minutes, or of 72°C and held for only 15 seconds will destroy disease-causing bacteria in milk, but may not completely destroy all organisms. Pasteurised milk is thus bacteriologically safe to drink, but will not keep for long at room temperature even in a conventionally sealed bottle or waxed-paper carton.

Fractionation

This consists in taking that part of a food which will keep and discarding the remainder. The obvious examples are butter and cheese. Butter is practically only the fat of milk, whereas cheese is a mixture of the chief milk protein, caseinogen together with the fat. Both will keep much longer than the milk from which they were derived. Part of the keeping quality is due to lactic acid, for the first stage in preparing both is to allow some decomposition, by bacteria, of the lactose of the milk, to this acid. In both butter and cheese, the keeping may be aided by adding salt. Cheeses may then also be smoked. Before the agricultural revolution of the late seventeenth and eighteenth centuries in Britain, cheese was a main dietary staple, along with bread, of the bulk of the population. Once again, it was a case of preserving as much as possible of the food content of the cow's milk, to use in a period when, owing to fodder shortage, the cow ceased her milk production.

Alcoholic fermentation could be regarded as a sort of fractionation. Up to 90% of the energy value of the starch in barley (beer) or of the sugar in grapes (wine) is preserved when these carbohydrates are converted by yeasts into *ethanol* (common or ethyl alcohol). Ethanol is toxic to almost all other micro-organisms, so the fermented barley *wort* or grape juice *must* will keep for weeks or years—as long as gastronomic taste or economics allows. Fermentation has been applied to cow's or to mare's milk in some parts of the world, to preserving cabbage (sauerkraut) and to various animal feedstuffs as silage.

The pros and cons of food processing

These may be considered under the headings gastronomic, dietetic and sociological or economic. As in the discussion on cooking, it is essential to consider factual evidence and not opinions or prejudices in this matter. While some losses in nutritional value or palatability may occur, these must be weighed against the gains in availability of out-of-season foods, foods from distant sources and the long-term offsetting periods of poor production due to climatic or other factors.

Gastronomic factors

In the majority of cases, the preservative methods alter the flavour or texture of a food for the worse. Mackerel that goes off the hook into the frying-pan is better than the same fish chilled for 24 hours in crushed ice, and far better than if it has hung around at normal temperatures for that time. Fresh fruit and vegetables from the garden are better than frozen, canned, salted or dried preparations. And so on. Perhaps cheese and wine are rareties which improve on keeping. Of course, conditioning plays a part in our responses to this matter. Canned or 'processed' peas may be preferred to frozen or fresh peas, because one has been accustomed from childhood to the preserved product and the fresh peas are a new food for which one has no acquired taste.

Dietetic factors

Preservative methods do little or no damage to the protein, fat or carbohydrate content of foods, nor is there any loss in inorganic materials. It is only among the vitamins that loss can occur. Ascorbic acid is decreased in canning and drying of fruits and vegetables, though in some quick-frozen preparations there may be more ascorbic acid than in fresh foods bought in the market and prepared at home. Riboflavine and nicotinic acid withstand processing, but thiamine may be lost by the heat treatment, or it may be leached out. The various things that happen to these vitamins in the processing of various grains to make them fit to eat have already been described and will not be considered again here.

Processing does often lower some of the value of the foods, but so long as we know how far, for example, the destruction of ascorbic acid has gone, we can obviate this loss. In any case, green vegetables or fruit with *reduced* vitamin content must be better than no foods with any vitamins at all.

Sociological and economic factors

Some processing of foods is inevitable in a highly organised urban industrial society. Town dwellers must be fed on foods transported some distance from where it is produced, and this food must be as wholesome after distribution as when it was produced. To cope with seasonal production, food may have to be brought from one side of the world to the other or stored for many months at a time. Finally, to counteract the effects of longer term climatic alterations, producing seasons of surplus or scarcity, preservation by one means or another enables the surpluses to be saved to cover times when foods are in short supply. At the present time, in the 1970s, although we have knowledge of the techniques necessary, national economic policies have prevented the establishment of such a 'world food bank' as was envisaged in the previous sentence. As I said in the beginning of this book, one of my few prejudices is the one of believing that every person has a right to an optimal diet and that economic and political power should not be used to prevent this right. In the short term, while resources of energy and fertilisers exist, with the known food production and preservative techniques, sufficient food *could* be produced and distributed to ensure that no person on the Earth had a less than adequate diet. The longer term future, with an expanding population and diminishing natural resources, is completely unknowable, but it is certain that without the level of international co-operation needed to achieve the short-term level of adequacy, the long-term problems will defeat the human race and widespread famine will ensue. These final glances at the present and future of global human nutrition are just as much part of the subject of human nutrition as is knowing what to buy at the supermarket in order to have a satisfactory meal at home tomorrow.

References

Connington, J. J. (1925) *Nordenholt's Million*. Republished by Penguin Books in 1946.

Department of Health and Social Security (1969) Report Public Health. Med. Subj. 120 and 122.

Duggan, A. (1959) *Knight with Armour*. Penguin Books. Originally published in 1950 by Faber.

McCance, R. A. & Widdowson, E. M. (1967) *The Composition of Foods*. Medical Research Council Special report series no. 297. HMSO.

National Academy of Sciences, USA (1974) *Recommended Daily Dietary Allowances*.

Oppé, T. E. *et al.* (1974) *Present-day practice in infant feeding*. HMSO.

Widdowson, E. M. (1936) A study of English diets by the individual method. 1 Men. *Journal of Hygiene* **36**, 269–292.

Widdowson, E. M. (1947) A study of individual children's diets. Medical Research Council Special Report Series 257. HMSO, London.

Widdowson, E. M. & McCance, R. A. (1936) A study of English diets by the individual methods. 2 Women. *Journal of Hygiene* **36**, 293–309.

Widdowson, E. M. & Thrussell, L. A. (1951) Medical Research Council Special report series no. 275. HMSO.

Zuntz, N. (1897) *Pflugers Arch ges Physiol*. **68**. 191.

Index

Index